Moira D. Shannon, EdD, RN

Long Term Care of the Aging

George Mason University Series, "Long-Term Care in Nursing"

Editors:

Moira Shannon, RN, EdD
Associate Professor

and

Rita M. Carty, DNSc, RN
Chairman

Department of Nursing, George Mason University
Fairfax, Virginia

Copyright 1984 by SLACK Incorporated

Printed in the United States of America

Library of Congress Catalog Card Number: 82-62399

ISBN: 0-943432-00-6

Published by:

SLACK Incorporated
6900 Grove Road
Thorofare, New Jersey 08086

Last digit is print number: 8 7 6 5 4 3 2 1

*F*OREWORD

AS FACULTY MEMBERS INVOLVED in the development and implementation of the Long-Term Care Nursing major in the graduate program at George Mason University, we became aware of the need for a series of monographs that would present a nursing perspective of some common topics relevant to long-term care across the life span. In an effort to meet this need, we have begun the preparation of a Long-Term Care Monograph Series that will extend over three years and include ten monographs, each designed to reflect the state of the art in the care and management of persons with long-term health concerns. These will provide a basis for education, practice and research in nursing.

The first monograph of the series is focused on long-term care of the aging. Other topics currently being developed include long-term care of persons with chronic illnesses such as cardiovascular, pulmonary and depressive problems, cancer, arthritis, alcoholism and diabetes. The managerial and administrative functions of nurses in long-term care facilities will also be developed.

Nurses face the challenge of being the nation's number one provider of health care services to individuals and families in the home, community or hospital. Preparation of nurses in long-term care across the life span has become one of the leading challenges facing nursing education today. This challenge involves a change in attitude away from curative measures to restorative measures with emphasis being placed on health promotion and disease prevention. As nurse educators, we welcome this challenge and are committed to increasing the body of knowledge on which nurses base their practice. To that purpose we dedicate this monograph series.

Moira Shannon
Rita M. Carty
(Series co-editors)
1984

PREFACE

THE PURPOSE OF THIS monograph is to provide an overview of gerontological nursing and related factors that impact on the health of the elderly in the United States. It is written for practicing registered nurses and nursing students who are interested in the care of the elderly. It may also be useful for practitioners in related health disciplines and others who work with and share concerns about the elderly.

Although nurses have always cared for elderly persons, basic curricula in nursing education in the past have not usually focused on the specific knowledge, attitudes and skills needed to better meet the developmental needs of elderly persons. This is done for other age groups that need special consideration such as children and adolescents. This monograph provides an overview of this knowledge and some of the attitudes reflected in practice and in the available literature on gerontological nursing.

The elderly person is an individual with identifiable developmental, physical, and psychosocial needs and resources. Although there is a high incidence of chronic disease among the elderly, they have many strengths and these can be used to promote and maintain health. The elderly person exists in the context of his personal and societal environment which includes his family and the community in which he lives. These influences must be considered in planning health care.

Chapter I discusses the professional implications of gerontological nursing with emphasis on standards and ethics as developed by the American Nurses Association. Chapter II identifies some of the theories on which gerontological nursing practice is based. Chapter III describes factors that contribute to healthy aging with an emphasis on health promotion and activities that assist in health maintenance. Chapter IV describes the changes that commonly occur in aging and some of the diseases that may accompany increasing longevity. Chapter V describes some of the support systems that assist elderly persons to maintain health and cope with illness. Chapter VI identifies the nursing process used to implement gerontological nursing care.

Suggested readings are included at the end of each chapter as guidelines for further reading on the topics introduced in the chapters.

Acknowledgments: I want to acknowledge the contributions of those who have helped to make this monograph a reality. The past and present staff of SLACK Incorporated have supported and encouraged this series of monographs. My co-editor for this series of monographs, Rita M. Carty, provided administrative as well as editorial assistance in the writing of this monograph. Mary C. Silva and Catherine Kopac reviewed the initial draft and gave constructive suggestions on revisions. Carol Panicucci reviewed the completed manuscript, raised critical questions and provided additional references and suggestions that strengthened the final version. The graduate students in Long Term Care/Gerontological Nursing at George Mason University stimulated many of the ideas presented as did my colleagues in nursing in many parts of the country.

To all of the above I am deeply grateful and special thanks go to my family and friends who provided ongoing personal support during the writing of this monograph.

MOIRA SHANNON

CONTENTS

INTRODUCTION

THE IMPETUS FOR A Long-Term Care Monograph Series grew out of the commitment of the faculty of the Department of Nursing, George Mason University, to address the issue of long-term care health problems across the life span.

The Department of Nursing initiated a new, non-traditional masters in nursing program in the later 1970's, including a clinical major in Long-Term Care Nursing. This innovative major was one of the first in the country. This is significant in that this focus preceded the current emphasis on chronic health care research and illness generated from studies such as the Institute of Medicine's 1983 study on nursing and nursing education. The IOM study strongly supports advanced nursing education to prepare for the care of the chronically ill.

The Long-Term Care Nursing curriculum at George Mason University includes major concepts related to health promotion, psycho-social and physical health assessment, chronic illness, rehabilitation, aging, health education, family and group theory, community resources, standards of advanced nursing practice and evaluation. Students may concentrate on any age group or chronic illness for practice and research. This nursing major recognizes the need for advanced nursing education in the care of individuals with chronic illness. Nurses have long been responsible for the care of these individuals and families in the home, community and health care settings. The current identification of a need for education, practice and research in long-term care nursing has produced the concurrent identification of a scarcity in the resources available for this care and a challenge to nursing to articulate the state of the art as it exists within our profession.

This Long-Term Care Monograph Series is one attempt at articulating the state of the art and providing theoretical foundations for nursing care of individuals with long-term care health problems in whatever setting they are found.

Nurse clinicians, clinical nurse specialists and nurse faculty members will contribute to this series. Many of these authors will be associated with George Mason University. Others will be nurses currently practicing long-term care nursing in various areas of our country who wish to share their knowledge and expertise via this monograph series.

The Department of Nursing, George Mason University, is committed to making this monograph series responsive to the needs of all nurses concerned with long-term care nursing, be that concern in practice, education or research.

Rita M. Carty, DNSc, RN
Chairman, Department of Nursing
George Mason University

1

Gerontological Nursing Practice

WHAT IS GERONTOLOGY?

The field of gerontology encompasses many disciplines and professions. In contrast to the geriatric orientation which focuses on diseases common to the elderly, gerontology focuses on the study of the aging process including behavioral, biological, psychological and social sciences; clinical practice; politics and policy; education; and research.

WHAT IS GERONTOLOGICAL NURSING PRACTICE?

In professional nursing practice, the American Nurses Association has defined five areas of clinical practice. These divisions of nursing practice are: psychiatric and mental health, community health, maternal and child health, medical-surgical, and gerontological. Of these five practice areas, all except maternal and child health include the elderly among their clients. However, it is the Division on Gerontological Nursing Practice that assumes leadership and responsibility for nursing care that is focused on specific health needs of the elderly.

A definition of Gerontological Nursing does not sound unique since it includes the same basic concepts used in nursing practice in all populations. It includes the process of assessing health status, making a nursing diagnosis, planning and implementing needed nursing and health care and evaluating the outcomes as a basis for continuing assessment. As in other areas of nursing, there is a focus on promoting and maintaining health, preventing and controlling disease, rehabilitating and restoring health and assisting in the process of dying.

The ANA standards of Gerontological Nursing Practice (1976) are in Appendix I. These standards can serve as a basis for evaluating both nursing care and administrative support for providing that care in agencies and institutions serving the elderly. The standards need to be easily accessible to nursing staff and are an important focal point for inservice education.

In addition to their use in guiding nursing practice in the care of the elderly, these standards are useful documents in educating administrators and others responsible for patient care about what constitutes nursing practice. This information must be shared to enable nurses to negotiate for needed support and an equitable share of available resources.

Another set of guidelines used to define nursing practice are those outlined in the Code of Ethics for Nurses (1976), which are in Appendix II. This code, like the standards of practice, serves as a guideline for nursing practice and needs the support of both nurses and administrators who have decision-making power.

In addition to providing guidelines for practice, the American Nurses Association has also developed recognition for advanced levels of practice through the process of certification. This provides documented evidence of demonstrated special qualifications to provide professional nursing care in defined areas of practice such as in Gerontology. Basic certification is based on clinical practice, not educational preparation. Nichols and Hallburg (1982) have described the personal and professional characteristics of a group of nurses certified in gerontological nursing. This group gave evidence of professional commitment and personality characteristics that were consistent with leadership ability.

WHO PRACTICES GERONTOLOGICAL NURSING?

All registered nurses who care for elderly persons in their work are practicing gerontological nursing. The level and scope of practice is defined by the expertise and commitment of the nurses and the realities of the setting.

Gerontological nursing is practiced wherever nurses provide service to elderly clients. In addition to hospitals and acute care settings, this can be done in nursing homes, extended care facilities, clinics, homes, community agencies and in non-health settings where health educational needs of the elderly are met by nurses such as in community classrooms and continuing education settings.

Realities of these settings such as the identified needs of clients and populations can be balanced quite creatively with the competencies of existing nursing personnel.

The level of educational preparation for nurses in Gerontology varies from basic nursing preparation for licensure as a registered nurse through baccalaureate, master's and doctoral degrees. Nurse practitioners are prepared beyond the basic level with advanced skills in health assessment and clinical management, while clinical nurse specialists are prepared at the master's level with appropriate content depth and practice skill in their clinical area. Although most basic nursing programs now include basic health assessment skills and some basic content in gerontology, many nurses caring for the elderly were educated in the past when this content was not included. For this reason it is important that continuing education be available and encouraged to enable nurses to improve their skills in providing care to the elderly. Such programs are best offered by nurses who are qualified not only in gerontological nursing content and skill but also in educational methodology. Administrative support for this type of education is essential to the quality of patient care.

WHY IS GERONTOLOGICAL NURSING PRACTICED?

The "why" for gerontological nursing practice is concerned more with "who needs it" than with "who does it." Assessment of need for this nursing service is found in the current demographic data which indicates that one of every nine persons in the United States today is elderly (over 65) and that life expectancy beyond that is 14 years for men and 18 years for women. These increased years have some limitations in respect to the quality of life and health. Sixty percent of the population over 85 years of age report functional difficulties and over 30 percent of this group are unable to manage the activities of daily living (Federal Council on the Aging, 1981).

Retirement usually lowers available income for the elderly thus limiting financial options. Normal aging contributes to a slowing down of physical processes and is often accompanied by gradual sensory losses such as sight and hearing. Chronic illness increases with age. Arthritis, hearing impairments and heart disease are the most common illnesses in the non-institutionalized elderly.

All of these changes present challenges to the elderly and usually necessitate additional support from family, friends and health professionals including nurses. Competent and caring practice of gerontological nursing can and does assist the elderly in meeting their health care needs. Having addressed the "who needs it" aspect of the "why" question, a brief comment on the "who does it" part of this question seems in order. Increasing numbers of nurses are caring for the elderly simply because they are there and need nursing care. What is exciting to those of us in gerontological nursing is that so many of these nurses, given adequate preparation and job support, are finding that they like it! And this, for them, has become the "why".

References

American Nurses' Association Division on Gerontological Nursing Practice. *Standards of Gerontological Nursing Practice.* Kansas City, MO: The Association, 1976.

American Nurses Association. *Code for Nurses with Interpretive Statements.* Kansas City, MO, 1976.

Federal Council on the Aging. *The Need for Long-Term Care: Information and Issues.* (DHHS Publication No. COHDS-81-20704). Washington, DC: U.S. Government Printing Office, 1981, 2.

House of Representatives Select Committee on Aging. *Every Ninth American* (1982 edition). Washington, DC: U.S. Government Printing Office, 1982.

Nichols, E. and Hallburg, J. Who are the certified gerontological nurses? *Journal of Gerontological Nursing.* November 1982, *8* (11), 618-622.

Suggested Readings on Gerontological Nursing Practice

Aiken, L.H. Nursing priorities for the 1980's: Hospitals and nursing homes. *American Journal of Nursing,* 1981, *81*(2), 324-330.

Brimen, P.F. Past, present and future in gerontological nursing research. *Journal of Gerontological Nursing, 1979,* 5(6), 27-34.

Certification Catalogue. Kansas City, MO: American Nurses' Association, 1983.

Gunter, L.M. and Miller, J.C. Toward nursing gerontology. *Nursing Research,* 1977, *26*(3), 208-219.

Martinson, I. *Gerontological Nursing.* A statement submitted to the National Advisory Council on Aging, Bethesda, MD, October 1980.

Munhall, P. Nursing philosophy and nursing research: In apposition or opposition. *Nursing Research,* May/June 1982, *31*(3), 176-181.

Silva, M.C. Philosophy, science, theory: Interrelationships and implications for nursing research. *Image,* October 1977, *9,* 59-63.

Weitzel, E. In pursuit of ANA certification in gerontological nursing. *Journal of Gerontological Nursing,* 1980, *6,* 136-139.

2

Theoretical Foundations for Gerontological Nursing

T heory in gerontology has concerned itself with both the individual and the larger society. Growth and development issues are especially appropriate to the study of elderly persons who have arrived at old age by experiencing many earlier ages. Biological theories of aging focus on the study of physical aging and its variations in each individual. Theories of aging such as those highlighting disengagement, activity, and continuity include psychological and social dimensions. This chapter will summarize some of the common theories currently used as a basis for gerontological nursing practice. Suggested readings at the end of the chapter provide more detailed sources of relevant theory.

LIFE SPAN DEVELOPMENTAL THEORY

Developmental theorists view life as a series of stages usually with accompanying tasks for which the individual is responsible. Havighurst (1948) originally described a developmental task as one which "arises at or about a certain period in the life of the individual, successful achievement of which leads to his happiness and to success with later tasks, while failure leads to unhappiness in the individual, disapproval by the society, and difficulty with later tasks." (p. 21). As seen in Table 2.1, Havighurst at that time conceptualized seven life stages with the final stage of later maturity covering all ages beyond 55 years. He further described the tasks for persons in the later maturity stage as including: gaining respect through cooperatively adjusting to environment which is largely manipulated by others rather than by oneself; learning to accept decreased health and strength; adjusting to retirement, economic and social problems and to changed living conditions; accepting the loss of one's long-time associates; continuing social interests in a less active capacity; and meeting social and civic obligations. The passage of time since these tasks were described has not substantially changed their nature. The age at which they must be faced may be beyond fifty-five, but conversations with elderly persons today will echo of the tasks described by Havighurst.

Another well-known developmental theorist is Erik Erikson (1963) who outlined eight stages in a life cycle based on chronological age and identified a specific developmental task for each stage (Table II). The task for the elderly is called ego integrity, which challenges the individual to accept the past and

8

TABLE 2-1
Life stages according to Robert Havighurst (1948)

Life Stage	Approximate Chronological Age
1. Infancy	Birth - 3 years
2. Early Childhood	3 - 6 years
3. Middle Childhood	6 - 12 years
4. Adolescence	12 - 18 years
5. Young Adulthood	18 - 30 years
6. Middle Years	30 - 55 years
7. Later Maturity	over 55 years

TABLE 2-2
*Erikson's Stages of Psychosocial Development and
Key Developmental Tasks (1963)*

Age	Key Developmental Tasks
First year	Trust vs. mistrust
1 - 3 years	Autonomy vs. shame and doubt
3 - 5 years	Initiative vs. guilt
6 - 11 years	Industry vs. inferiority
12 - 16 years	Identity vs. role confusion
16 years to adulthood	Intimacy vs. isolation
Adulthood to late adulthood	Generativity vs. stagnation
Late adulthood	Integrity vs. despair and disgust

interpret it as meaningful. In this framework, failure to achieve this integrity would lead toward the negative direction of despair and disgust in which an individual would be unable to find meaning in life and accept its limitations. In considering the bipolar attributes described by Erikson, it is noted that the ideal is not seen at either end of the continuum of the task described but at a point in the direction of the positive.

Recent life stage categorizations are reflecting awareness that adulthood shares many phases and characteristics previously detailed only in childhood phases of development. Stevenson (1977) has described three stages of adult life by chronological age and has suggested major developmental tasks to be completed. In this framework for adulthood, middle adulthood is labeled middlescence I (30-50 years) and middlescence II (50-70 years) with identified tasks for the latter being to assume primary responsibility for continued survival of the nation. The late stage of adulthood (70 years +) is seen as the time for sharing the wisdom of age, reviewing life, and putting affairs in order.

Recent studies have raised questions about developmental models of adult life. Lacy and Hendricks (1980) were unable to support developmental stage models in their research. They suggest that the fluid nature of the adult years is not unidirectional or unitary and that development must be studied in a social context. Their findings indicated that sex, race, social class, historical period and cohorts were factors as relative to attitudes and perceptions as life cycle stages.

Developmental models and the concept of accompanying tasks do offer an organized way of thinking about aging. Further research is needed to evaluate developmental theory in relation to clinical practice.

DISENGAGEMENT THEORY

Disengagement theory is built on the premise that as people grow old they choose to withdraw from the world and become interested primarily in themselves. One of the pioneer efforts in disengagement theory was that of Cummings and Henry (1961) which described a disengagement process between the aged and society that was mutually accommodating. Later theoretical developments have questioned the mutuality of the disengagement process. A basic assumption of disengagement theory is that it is "natural" and good to withdraw from society. This withdrawal is seen as a norm, without consideration of individual differences and societal barriers that could contribute to differences in inclination toward and ability to achieve this withdrawal.

ACTIVITY THEORY

Activity theory conceptualizes that old age is an extension of middle age and thus activities of middle age should be continued to assure adaptation and adjustment. Havighurst, Neugarten and Tobin (1968) further suggested that substitute activities should be found for ones that must be relinquished. This includes substitutes for work after retirement and for relationships when those are lost.

This theory assumes an intrinsic value for both work and activity and does not distinguish the quality or quantity for either. It emphasizes the active and healthy aged but is less than satisfactory in application to the frail elderly and those who are most vulnerable by reason of their social status.

CONTINUITY THEORY

Neugarten, Havighurst and Tobin (1968) identified weaknesses in both disengagement and activity theory. They focused on a theory of aging that supported continuity of the individual personality with developmental implications. Their research indicated that older persons who had achieved a degree of integration had a high life satisfaction regardless of activity level.

Continuity theory focuses on the premise that as we age we tend to maintain the personality traits of our younger years and to adapt these as necessary rather than to adopt new ones. Neugarten (1977) has well described the relationships in research related to aging and personality. She has suggested the need for collaboration between theorists and clinicians and identified culture and history as inextricably bound to our approach in the study of aging.

Covey (1981) supports the scope of the continuity theory and its potential to incorporate the positive aspects of other major theories. This theory supports individual desires to hold on to roles that have been rewarding in the past.

Continuity as a characteristic of aging is questioned by Fox (1981-1982) who also doubts if it eases adaptive processes in late life. The possibility of continuity theory supporting a programmed approach to old age, with minimal motivation for positive change, is raised as a question.

BIOLOGIC THEORY OF AGING

Biology of aging is a field with many directions. Research efforts in rodents and other animal species are numerous and have served as a basis for hypothesizing on biological changes in aging humans. Finch and Hayflick (1977) have compiled an impressive collection of articles on the biology of aging which described the aging process at various levels including molecular, cellular, tissue and organ, and whole animal. Research is continuing in many of these areas with new and sometimes contradictory findings continuing to emerge.

Eliopoulos (1979) has simplified and summarized the most common biological theories into five categories:

1. Autoimmune theory describes aging as the result of various body systems beginning to reject their own tissues.
2. Wear and tear theory describes the end result of an organism's stress as cumulative with the end result of accumulated stress being death.
3. Metabolic waste theory focuses on the accumulated wastes that develop during aging which eventually cause dysfunction.
4. Mutation theory examines how agents cause a change in the DNA molecule, thus changing how the DNA is able to express itself.
5. Biological clock theory describes how each cell is preprogrammed within DNA to a specific life expectancy.

Finch and Severson (1981) raise incisive questions about current theories of biologic aging and the attitudes which flow from them. They question that aging is necessarily a degenerative and deteriorating process that is intrinsic to every cell and suggest that it is a selective process varying from one individual to another and from one system to another within the individual. They suggest that a dominance of the physiological mechanisms that involve neuroendocrine-control mechanisms and hormones may exist at specific stages of aging followed in later stages of aging by time-dependent changes such as aging-pigment accumulation or mutation. These authors further elaborate on the negative effects of belief in biologic theory that deny that certain parts of the human body have the capacity for normal functioning even in advanced age.

NURSING IMPLICATIONS FROM THEORY

What is the meaning of theory to the nurse caring for elderly individuals? A theory is not an absolute truth. It is an intellectual process aimed at discovering truth, and it can be used to connect various concepts in a specific way that allows for development and testing. It is a common stereotype to assume that nurses primarily in education and research lack a "real world" touch. It is an equally common assumption that the nurse at the bedside is primarily practicing at a technical level with little theoretical foundation. Fortunately, the increasing level of education of many nurses, and the increasing level of clinical skill within educational processes, has softened the old stereotypes and sound practice based on theory is becoming more widespread. For the gerontological nurse, incorporating theory into clinical practice provides support for creative therapeutic care to the elderly rather than a primary focus on custodial care.

All theory development requires ongoing testing for validity and reliability. As we use supportive theories from other disciplines such as biology, psychology, sociology and others, nurses must be selective in terms of which theories are appropriate to specific practice, and critical in the effectiveness of the theories chosen. Exchange of information that will contribute to this effort must be interdisciplinary and represent the collaboration of both scientists and clinicians in nursing.

Theories on aging provide the basis for individualized assessments of behavior. An example of this using growth and development theory would be to recognize despair in comments about how a person has spent his life. The nurse caring for an elderly person who is making such comments would recognize that there was a lack of the desired ego integrity at this stage in life. Interventions could be directed toward assisting the person with the life review process as described by Butler and Lewis (1982) in an effort to assist with integration of life events.

Personality and continuity theory can offer a conceptual basis for deciding if an elderly person's withdrawal from activities and relationships is a lifelong coping pattern or a reaction to external circumstances beyond his control that make activity and personal communication difficult. Nursing intervention in such a situation could aim for positive changes in the person's environment and social support system.

SUMMARY

This chapter has provided an overview of current theories foundational to gerontological nursing practice. Developmental, biological, and psychosocial theories have been briefly described. The need for continued theory development and evaluation as a foundation for gerontological nursing practice is emphasized. The interdisciplinary focus of gerontology further necessitates that theory development and evaluation be collaborative between the many disciplines concerned with the process of aging.

References

Butler, R. and Lewis, M. *Aging and mental health* (3rd ed.). St. Louis: C.V. Mosby Co., 1982.

Covey, H. A reconceptualization of continuity theory: Some preliminary thoughts. *The Gerontologist*, 1981, *21*, 629-633.

Cummings, E. and Henry, W.E. Growing old: The process of disengagement. New York: Basic Books, 1961.

Eliopoulos, C. *Gerontological nursing*. New York: Harper and Row, 1979.

Erikson, E.H. *Childhood and society* (2nd ed.). New York: W.W. Norton, 1963.

Finch, C.E. and Hayflick, L. (Eds.) *Handbook of the biology of aging*. New York: Van Nostrand Reinhold Co., 1977.

Finch, C.E. and Severson, J.A. Biological theories of aging. In Irene M. Burnside, *Nursing and the aged*. New York: McGraw-Hill Book Co., 1981.

Fox, J. Perspectives on the continuity perspective. *International Journal of Aging and Human Development*, 1981-82, *14*, 97-115.

Havighurst, R.J. *Developmental tasks and education*. New York: McKay, 1948.

Havighurst, R., Neugarten, B. and Tobin, S. Disengagement and patterns of aging. In B. Neugarten (Ed.), *Middle age and aging*. Chicago: The University of Chicago Press, 1968.

Lacy, Wm.B. and Hendricks, J. Developmental models of adult life: Myth or reality. *International Journal of Aging and Human Development*, 1980, *11*(2), 89-110.

Neugarten, B.L. Personality and aging. In James Birren, and K. Warner Schaie (Eds.), *The Psychology of Aging*. New York: Van Nostrand Reinhold Co., 1977.

Stevenson, J.S. *Issues and crises during middlescence*. New York: Appleton-Century-Crofts, 1977.

Suggested Readings on Theoretical Foundations for Gerontological Nursing

Atchley, R.C. *The social forces in later life*. Belmont, CA: Wadsworth Publishing Co., 1980.

Bandura, A. *Social learning theory*. Englewood Cliffs, NJ: Prentice-Hall, Inc., 1977.

Binstock, R.N. and Shanas, E. *The handbook of aging and the social sciences*. New York: Van Nostrand Reinhold Co., 1976.

Birren, J.E. and Schaie, K.W. *The handbook of the psychology of aging*. New York: Van Nostrand Reinhold Co., 1977.

Fisk, M. Tasks and crises of the second half of life: The interrelationship of commitment, coping and adaptation. In J.E. Birren & R.B. Sloane (Eds.), *Handbook of Mental Health and Aging*. Englewood Cliffs, NJ: Prentice-Hall, 1980, 337-373.

Havighurst, R.J. *Developmental Tasks and Education* (3rd ed.). New York: McKay, 1972.

Levinson, D.J. *The Seasons of a Man's Life*. New York: Ballantine Books, 1978.

Longino, C. and Kart, C. Explicating activity theory: A formal replication. *Journal of Gerontology*, 1982, *37*, 713-722.

Lowenthal, M.F., and Chiriboga, D. Social stress and adaptation: Toward a life course perspective. In C. Eisdorfer and M.P. Lawton (Eds.), *The psychology of adult development and aging*. Washington, DC: American Psychological Association, 1973.

Maslow, A.H. *Motivation and personality*. New York: Harper and Row, 1954.

Neugarten, B.L. (Ed.) *Middle age and aging* (5th pub.). Chicago: University of Chicago Press, 1975.

Neugarten, B. Time, age and the life cycle. *American Journal of Psychiatry*, July 1979, *136*(7), 887-894.

Panicucci, C.L. Developmental patterns of interaction. In D.A. Jones, C.F. Denbar, and M.M. Jirovic (Eds.), *Medical-Surgical Nursing*. New York: McGraw-Hill, 1978, 82-88.

Pearlin, L.I. and Schooler, C. The structure of coping. *Journal of Health and Social Behavior*, 1978, *19*, 2-21.

Reff, M.E. and Schneider, E.L. (Eds.). *Biological Markers of Aging*. Washington, DC, NIH, 1982. (NIH # 82-2221).

Riley, M.W., Abeles, R.P., and Teitelbaum, M.S. *Aging from birth to death*. Vol. II: Sociotemporal Perspectives 1982. Boulder, CO: Westview Press, Inc.

Rockstein, M. and Sussman, M. *Biology of aging*. Belmont, CA: Wadsworth Publishing Co., 1979.

Schaie, K.W. and Geiwitz, J. *Adult development and aging*. Boston: Little, Brown and Co., 1982.

Watson, W. *Aging and social behavior*. Belmont, CA: Wadsworth Health Sciences Division, 1982.

3

Promotion and Maintenance of Health in the Aging Process

Today's concept of health care includes not only the prevention and treatment of disease but also the promotion of positive health often referred to as wellness. This requires public support as well as the efforts of individuals and health care professionals. Nurses are faced with the challenge of strengthening their interventions for health promotion. This includes a strong commitment to health education and patient education. The nurse can encourage behavioral changes that contribute to wellness in caring for elderly persons. These include good nutritional habits, physical fitness, stress management, and healthy sexual attitudes. Environmental factors are essential to achieving health. Since elderly persons often perceive a diminishing control over their environment, it is important that those who assume responsibility for the care of the elderly are aware of the relationships between environment and health. Financial constraints, such as the fact that Medicare does not pay for health maintenance activities, must be recognized. This chapter will discuss the topics mentioned above as they impact on the health care of the elderly.

PUBLIC SUPPORT FOR HEALTH

One of the major governmental efforts to promote health and prevent disease was the publication of "Healthy People" - the Surgeon General's report on health promotion and disease prevention published in 1979. This work established our strategies for health in this country, identified the major health problems, and described current disease prevention measures. This report identified five measurable and achievable public health goals, one for each identified age group in this society. The goal focusing on healthy older adults was: "To improve the health and quality of life for older adults and, by 1990, to reduce the average annual number of days of restricted activity due to acute and chronic conditions by 20 percent, to fewer than 30 per year for people aged 65 and older" (p. 71). This report stated that 80 percent of older Americans have one or more chronic conditions and that 30 percent of national health care expenditures were spent on medical treatment for this age group. The specific subgoals in this report were:

1. to increase the number of older adults who can function independently, and

2. to reduce premature death from influenza and pneumonia.

The fact that only five percent of older persons reside in institutions was emphasized, with most older people living in their own homes either alone, with a spouse or with others. However, 45 percent have activity limitations - some due to mental disabilities, but the majority due to the physical handicaps of heart disease, arthritis and rheumatism, hearing loss and visual problems.

Suggested strategies to increase independent functioning in this group included outreach programs to locate those who need assistance, geriatric screening programs, and community based comprehensive health services preferably provided at one center. The development of vaccines for both influenza and pneumonia offer promise of reducing the death rate due to these diseases.

Needed health related activities to respond to identified health concerns were grouped into the following categories:

1. *Preventive health services* - services delivered to individuals by health care providers to reduce the risk of specific disease,
2. *Health protection* - measures which governmental and other agencies and industry can use to protect persons from hazards, and
3. *Health promotion* - those activities which can be used by individuals and communities to promote healthy lifestyles.

The 15 priority areas identified under the three sections described above are listed below with an asterisk used to designate those areas that are most relevant to the elderly.

Preventive Health Services

* High blood pressure control
  Family planning
  Pregnancy and infant health
  Immunization
  Sexually transmitted diseases

Health Protection

  Toxic agent control
  Occupational safety and health
* Accident prevention and injury control
  Fluoridation and dental health
  Surveillance and control of infectious diseases

Health Promotion

  Smoking and health
* Misuse of alcohol and drugs
* Nutrition
* Physical fitness and exercise
* Control of stress and violent behavior

In 1980, a follow-up document to "Healthy People" was published entitled "Promoting Health/Preventing Disease". This report described specific objectives for each of the 15 priority areas previously identified and all of these objectives were seen as the objectives for the nation of 1990. For each of the health priority areas, review of the following factors was included:

Nature and extent of the problem

Prevention/promotion measures

Specific objectives for 1990 or earlier

Principal assumptions, and

Data sources

The recommendations based on these reports are beginning to be implemented in health care in general, and are included in the care of gerontological clients.

At the 1981 White House Conference on Aging, the report of the Technical Committee on Health Maintenance and Health Promotion focused on three major areas:

1. Health Maintenance and Health Promotion Services
2. Behavioral issues in Health Maintenance and Health Promotion
3. Special issues in Health Maintenance and Health Promotion

All three of these areas are of concern to the nursing profession. This report discussed service implications for physical and social environments; physical, mental and dental health; rehabilitation; linkages; and cost reimbursement. Behavioral issues in health education, nutrition, stress management, and drug and alcohol related problems were described with identification of older Americans as a resource and suggestions for self care and mutual help. Special issues including distinct populations of elderly such as rural, minority and women were identified. Research needs related to health maintenance and health promotion in the elderly were noted.

These efforts on the part of the federal government to assess and plan for the health of the elderly in this country are an encouraging beginning. The implementation and evaluation of these programs will be the responsibility not only of the government but also of the private sector and especially of the health professionals including nurses who are committed to the care of persons of all ages.

In considering the federal categories of health concerns, health protection is aimed at population groups and is primarily the concern of federal, state and local government with input from the private sector. Preventive health services are provided to individuals by medical and other health care practitioners and are aimed at preventing and controlling disease. The health promotion focus is on assisting individuals to improve their health by influencing lifestyle behaviors. Health is promoted through the process of health education and the goal of health education is to move people away from illness toward the concept of wellness.

HEALTH EDUCATION

Health education is defined as any combination of learning opportunities designed to facilitate voluntary adaptations of behavior conducive to health. Patient education is the process of health education applied to persons who are currently receiving medical treatment to manage an illness.

There is an implied assumption in health education that if people are informed about constructive behavior alternatives that will increase their level of health, and given motivation and assistance in making these changes, they will change their behavior. This is the rationale for spending human and material resources on health education, but evaluation is needed to validate the outcome before the process is complete. The nurse who shares with her client how they will jointly evaluate results in relation to the person's health has taken a giant step towards sound evaluation of the health education process. It is important to remember that health education is an appropriate intervention only for those situations that are controlled by behavior. This is the primary difference between information sharing and health education. It may add to a patient's knowledge to share information about a genetic condition that affects health but since the person usually cannot change genetic traits by changing behavior, such information shared cannot achieve the desired outcome of health education, i.e. to effect through learning a voluntary behavior change that is conducive to improved health.

The patient's Bill of Rights, developed in 1972, identified education as the right of all patients in hospitals. Assuring this right for elderly persons means making any needed adaptations to enable them to take part in the health care process. This means assessing learning ability, existing knowledge base about the topic, motivation and skill in carrying out desired changes.

One way to assist learning for elderly persons would be to give them a written handout, in large print, using non-glare paper at the time of instruction. They could then use this written material to reinforce what has been taught. It also helps to ask how they have been able to make needed changes in their past lives. If they can identify how they do this successfully, they provide clues about their strengths and individuality which will help in effective planning.

Although health and patient education is a recognized function of nursing, there are some pitfalls inherent in past nursing education that need to be recognized. Nursing is often oriented to treatment of disease in persons who are patients in a hospital or other constrained environment and who see the nurse as responsible for their care under orders from their doctor. Health education is oriented to a learning process in persons who may not be directly under the care of a doctor, who have control over their living environment and the choices they make, and who see themselves as ultimately responsible for their behavior and their health. Shine, Silva and Weed (1983) have described knowledge and skills in health education seen as needed in a baccalaureate nursing program.

The nurse who has not yet developed the skills of health education needs to allow time and opportunity to learn them. By expanding the repertoire of skills, the nurse can broaden clinical practice to include health promotion and health education functions as well as those nursing interventions traditionally used in the care of the aged. This type of expansion reflects a philosophy of intervention that may be closer to that of health education than that of more traditional medical and nursing services, but it is important to health promotion in the elderly.

Nurses responsible for health promotion need knowledge about existing public and private resources that enhance care of the elderly. The American Hospital Association in Chicago has a center for health promotion that provides consumer health information for all ages.

Specific to health information for elderly persons is the "Age Page" published regularly by the National Institute on Aging and available free on request. These publications provide information about a variety of topics such as skin care, arthritis, urinary incontinence, constipation and many others. The information is clear, concise and summarizes not only possible causes for the conditions but also suggested remedies. The education divisions of large pharmaceutical companies provide information booklets on health concerns for the elderly such as nutrition, stress management and others.

WELLNESS

The concept of wellness was publicized in 1961 by Halbert Dunn in his book called *High Level Wellness*. Many others have elaborated on this with one of the most common illustrations being that of a continuum with illness and premature death at one end and wellness at the other.

(Figure 3-1)

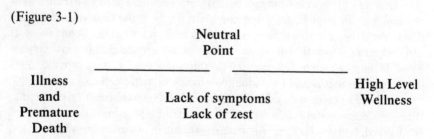

On this continuum, an individual could be located at different levels depending on physical and psychosocial health factors. The important indicators of health would be whether the general direction was towards wellness or illness.

A concept similar to wellness, and often used in conjunction with wellness practice, is that of self actualization as described by Maslow (1954). Self actualization was seen as the high point of a hierarchy of human needs. These include physiologic needs; safety and security; love and belonging; and self esteem self-actualization. The physiological needs include food and water, air, rest, elimination and freedom from pain, wherever a person is living. Safety and security needs range from the threat of crimes of violence and theft to the comfort needs of a shelter.

The need for love and belonging describes meaningful relationships with other people who can provide approval, affection and appropriate touching. Esteem includes self esteem and self identity as well as the esteem of others. The zenith of Maslow's hierarchy of needs, self actualization, is the maximizing of an individual's potential in life, and could be one of the joys of old age.

Our health care system has many advanced tools for diagnosing illness but lacks a similar sophistication in identifying wellness. This could be due to the fact that part of wellness lies in the individual's perception of how he feels. For the elderly person, a sense of wellness and a maximization of existing potential may coexist with some of the infirmities of aging. The following case study demonstrates how this can complicate communication between the person and those who are helping him to care for himself.

Mr. A is a 76-year-old man and was recently hospitalized with a ruptured colon due to diverticulitis. Following surgery, which included a temporary colostomy, Mr. A had done well and was ready for discharge with the long-term plan being to close the colostomy and reconnect the bowel in 6 months. Prior to this illness episode, Mr. A was considered well. A widower for 15 years, he lived alone in his own house in a community where he had lived for almost 50 years. His only daughter and her family lived in another state, and although they spoke often by phone and visited two or three times each year, Mr. A perceived himself as alone and responsible for his own health and well-being - a responsibility that he welcomed and felt quite capable of handling.

Prior to the discharge planning meeting, the nurse spoke with both Mr. A and his daughter who was visiting to validate their perceptions of what the convalescence period would mean. The physician had suggested that at his age, Mr. A might want to consider living in an extended care facility until his colostomy could be closed and his status could then be evaluated. This suggestion was supported by others on the discharge planning team as it was assumed that such an arrangement would minimize the possibility of complications and would assure nutrition and colostomy care for this period of time.

Using an approach of listening before suggesting alternatives, the nurse asked Mr. A and his daughter what they were thinking. Mr. A, who had always been strong in his opinions and independent in his functioning, envisioned himself living as he always had with the single added chore of caring for the colostomy and perhaps getting a little extra rest after his ordeal in the hospital. His daughter, Mrs. L, was not totally comfortable with this arrangement, feeling that her father should have some kind of additional support during the months ahead. Further questioning revealed that this feeling had existed prior to the recent illness since Mrs. L had read and heard so many things about the loneliness of the aged and was feeling somewhat guilty about living so far from her father as he was growing old. When the nurse then suggested the plan of moving into a nursing home or extended care facility for several months, Mrs. L looked relieved. Mr. A looked appalled. His first question was WHY? Unable to think of a satisfactory answer on the spot, the nurse explained that they were only brainstorming all the possibilities and that the whys needed to be considered from positive and negative perspectives for all the alternatives presented.

Surprised and uneasy about Mr. A's response and her own inability to defend what she had thought sounded like a good solution to the problem, the nurse consulted with others on the team. After an open discussion that included an assessment of Mr. A's wellness needs and developmental status as well as his physical and psychosocial needs, the discharge planning nurse realized that she had fallen into a common trap. She had made the problem the center of the planning rather than the person. This is easy to do in a hospital situation where the main emphasis is on the problem, where staff is highly trained in the technology needed to provide medical and nursing treatments and where even the recording system is often organized around existing health problems. Without minimizing the importance of treating problems, it is also essential to keep them in perspective as they relate to the person. In the situation described above, the health professionals were looking at solutions of how they and other health care providers could best treat the problem.

Mr. A was looking at how he could best care for himself with his problem. His existing lifestyle met his needs as a person and this illness had altered only his bowel function. To alter his lifestyle would cause disruption and change in many areas of his life, thus creating additional stress that would need to be handled.

Mrs. L needed some reassurance that she was not being negligent toward her father by allowing him to maintain his former lifestyle since this was his choice and living alone does not necessarily mean being lonely at any age. The fact that Mr. A did not perceive himself as lonely and that his longtime friends and neighbors in the community functioned as an extended family network was a fact that had been validated. Both the nurse and Mrs. L needed to view the situation apart from their own biases that included dependency as a norm for all elderly.

The very real challenge of caring for a colostomy did need to be planned for but by viewing this as something to be dealt with within the context of what was a satisfactory living situation, rather than allowing it to overwhelm the living situation, normalcy and health became the focus rather than illness. The visiting nurse service was contacted and arrangements were made for regular visits to assist with colostomy care. The local homemaker service was able to provide assistance with the upkeep of the house for a few weeks while Mr. A regained his strength. Friends were contacted and asked to make at least one visit per day, to assure continued social contacts until Mr. A regained his strength and could go out and socialize as before.

In summary, Mr. A had a high level of wellness in his physical and mental health, had an adequate social support system, was financially secure and lived in an environment in which he could meet his basic needs independently. These strengths deserved support to assure his continued wellness.

NUTRITION

Good nutrition is one of the cornerstones of good health at any age. It is an essential component of curriculum in nursing education and nurses are often the health care provider with the most opportunity to teach and reinforce the teachings of other professionals such as the nutritionist.

As with other health related concepts, nutrition exists in a context of biological, physical and psychosocial factors that vary with each individual. Biological factors include the individual anatomical and physiological characteristics that affect a person's ability to ingest, digest, and absorb nutrients. Sensory losses in aging that affect taste and smell are special considerations. Physical factors are the types of food available, cooking and storing facilities, and the atmosphere in which the food is served and eaten. Psychosocial factors include the individual cultural and religious values as well as the economic capacity to purchase nutritious food.

As people age, their caloric requirements decrease although there is still need for high nutritional requirements. This situation creates the challenge to provide for needed nutriments on fewer calories.

One of the most common problems of nutrition in the elderly is that of people who live alone and don't want to "bother" with cooking meals just for themselves. It is important for the nurse who is counselling such a person to be aware of issues of self esteem, loneliness and dependency. The nutritional problem may be the symptom that expresses other concerns. Comfort (1976) described food as one of the lifelong pleasures. The elderly can enjoy this pleasure but often need supportive counselling to find alternative ways if the people with whom they once enjoyed meals are gone and/or their food budget has become limited in comparison to prior times.

PHYSICAL FITNESS

Physical fitness is a popular term in all age groups in the United States today. School children have regular exercise periods as an essential component of curriculum. This was not always true, and many elderly persons are not oriented toward or comfortable with the concept of regular physical exercise. The current trend toward physical fitness focuses on two distinct types of exercise: stretching or limbering of the body and aerobic exercises to strengthen the cardiovascular system. These combined with weight control, good nutrition and stress management are seen as the keys to physical fitness.

These cornerstones for health can be cultivated and encouraged in the elderly. Advocates of physical fitness are often responsible for convincing their peers of the resultant benefits. For the nurse working with the elderly, there is a two-fold approach. The first is role modeling by maintaining one's own physical fitness. The second is encouraging elderly people to begin whatever levels of exercise are available and appropriate to them as individuals regardless of age.

A current project relative to physical fitness and the elderly is being implemented through the Health Education Resource Center at George Mason University in Virginia. This project, called HEP, is aimed at promoting healthy lifestyle patterns among the well elderly in the community through physical exercises, thus reducing risk for the high incidence of chronic disease associated with aging.

Another project focused on health promotion for older adults is the Wallingford Wellness Project at the University of Washington in Seattle. Similar projects will continue to develop as both the elderly and society recognize the importance of health promotion.

STRESS MANAGEMENT

In the U.S. Department of Health and Human Services report on "Promoting Health/Preventing Disease" (1980), stress refers to "those pressures and tensions (whether behaviorally, biologically, economically or environmentally induced) which, unless suitably managed, can lead to psychological or physiological maladaptations manifested in phenomena such as fatigue, headache, obesity, absenteeism, illness, accident-proneness or violence" (p. 83). In forming objectives relative to the control of stress, this report specifically mentions the need for medical and nursing schools to offer instruction to help students understand the pathophysiology of stress and its management.

Selye (1975) defined stress as the wear and tear that a person experiences at a given point in time. The factor that causes the stress is seen as a stressor, and the individual's response is the stress reaction. The desired outcome when stress occurs is to be able to maintain a state of equilibrium by adapting. Failure to adapt can lead to tissue damage and altered functioning of organs.

For health practitioners who are concerned with health promotion, stress management is seen as essential before the appearance of overt signs and symptoms. Balanced nutrition and regular physical exercise contribute to a better level of general health and thus increase the biologic resources that will be available to an individual when stressors appear as they will. Relaxation exercises, meditation, yoga, music and dance are common activities that are used with elderly persons to reduce stress and promote positive attitudes and behaviors. When adverse stress reactions do occur, the nurse can assist elderly people by helping them identify the causes and delineate the available alternatives for managing the stressors.

SEXUALITY

Another aspect of an elderly person's being that contributes to positive health goals is healthy sexuality. Sexuality is a deep and pervasive aspect of the total human personality which includes feelings and behavior, not only as a sexual being, but also as a male or female (SEICUS, 1970). It is a treasured vehicle for sharing with others at any stage of the life cycle as well as an essential instinct for the survival of the human race.

For the elderly person, the reproductive aspect of sex is not usually a factor. Social values in some segments of society primarily value the reproductive function of sex and the older person who continues to enjoy sex beyond the reproductive years is considered somewhat perverse. Traditional values emphasize a heterosexual identity. Celibacy is accepted, especially if it is for an altruistic reason and is voluntarily embraced as in a religious vocation or in the chosen celibate state of married persons whose spouses are ill, dead or in absence for other reasons.

Homosexual identity is becoming acceptable to a larger portion of society as is masturbation and sexual relationships among non-married couples. The main indicators of the value of sex in the elderly will be their past experiences, their socialization on sexual values, the environment in which they are now living and the attitudes of the people close to them.

In recent years, persons dealing with the elderly have become increasingly aware of the variety of individual sexual differences. Films for educating the non-elderly in the care of their elders have brought stereotyped attitudes regarding sexuality of the elderly to new levels of awareness.

Butler and Lewis (1976) have described the common medical and emotional problems that affect sex in the elderly. They also identify solutions to these problems and emphasize the value of sex after the age of sixty. Common medical problems affecting sexual activities are those such as heart disease, stroke, diabetes, arthritis, anemia, backache, hernia, Parkinson's disease, stress incontinence, prostatitis and Peyronie's disease in men, and vaginal abnormalities in women. Surgical interventions that may require sexual adjustments include hysterectomy, mastectomy, prostatectomy, orchidectomy, colostomy and ileostomy. Common emotional problems that affect sex are problems in the relationship between the sexual partners, widowhood and grief, sexual guilt and shame, and for males - the fear of impotence.

Suggestions to improve on the general changes that occur in aging may affect sexual feeling. These include activities focused on maintaining general health and appearance through nutrition and exercise; having adequate rest and relaxation; improving personal appearance through cleanliness; care of the hair and skin; and wearing appropriate clothing. In addition to seeking medical attention for specific diseases and postoperative follow-up care, the elderly person may need to seek counselling on realistic expectations related to sexual functioning and acceptable alternatives that are compatible with existing illness. New patterns of lovemaking may be helpful to both partners. Support groups such as those for stroke patients and persons with ostomies can offer both support and new ideas on how to cope with sexual problems that arise.

The research of Masters and Johnson (1966) described some of the physiological changes with aging. Responses may slow down, but they do not necessarily disappear. With a supportive environment and a caring partner, most elderly persons can make needed adaptations in techniques to accommodate satisfactory sexual activity.

The female vagina may shorten and lose its elasticity and its capacity to lubricate on demand. Exercises can strengthen structural weakness and creative use of appropriate lubricants prior to sexual intercourse can solve the lubrication problem as a part of lovemaking. The male may take longer to achieve an erection but again this situation can be creatively handled during foreplay with a caring partner.

It is important for the nurse to understand the biological and psychosocial facts of sexuality in the aged, and to separate these from personal or societal attitudes if there is some discrepancy. McCarthy (1979) summarized the three major factors that influence geriatric sexuality as capacity, interest and opportunity. Nurses can often support the promotion and maintenance of all three and thus make a contribution to sexual health in the elderly. The following anecdote is an example of this.

Mr. S, a senior nursing student, was gravely concerned about what he had just seen. Mrs. B was his patient in the nursing home that day and after he had assisted her in her morning care and seen that she was comfortable in her wheelchair, he had gone to do his charting. His notebook was still in her room and thus he had returned to her room much earlier than she expected. As he approached the partially closed door (closing of doors was against the policy of the nursing home) he heard voices. One voice was clearly that of a man, not the doctor. He approached cautiously and, looking into the room, he saw Mr. W from the other wing of the nursing home sitting next to Mrs. B. She was eating bacon with one hand and holding onto his arm with the other. He was caressing her breast with his free hand and they both seemed to be enjoying the situation. The student was worried that Mrs. B was eating bacon since she was on a low salt diet and occasionally had difficulty with pitting edema in her ankles. He was aware that "fraternizing" was not allowed between patients at that point but this did not disturb him at all since he saw the rule as one that needed to be reexamined and followed with selectivity that did not negate the human needs of individuals.

The student later talked with Mrs. B and learned that her frequent early morning visits from Mr. W were one of the bright spots in her life. The visits began when these two people had met at a social event at the nursing home and Mrs. B had confided to Mr. W that she would do anything to be able to have an occasional piece of bacon but the staff would not allow this since it was not on her diet. The student asked Mrs. B if she would still want Mr. W to visit if she were able to get the bacon from another source. "Oh, yes!" she replied, "but I wouldn't want to let him know that. This way he thinks he is giving me something that nobody else can provide." "Is he?" asked the student. "Oh, yes," she replied, "but it isn't the bacon."

This situation illustrates an existing relationship between an elderly man and woman who are living in an institution and still enjoying one aspect of sexuality. It demonstrates the environmental constraints often found in institutions and raises questions of privacy, individual rights, agency policies, professional ethics and priorities in patient care. The answers to these questions are an ongoing challenge to practitioners and administrators in long-term care facilities.

ENVIRONMENT

The concept of environment encompasses biological, physical and psychosocial dimensions all of which impact on health. The main biological concern is organisms capable of spreading disease. Physical factors include climate, water supply, air quality, sanitation, space, housing, and food and water supplies. Psychosocial factors include laws, economic resources, health care delivery system, educational and recreational opportunities and general attitudes of society toward its aging population. A general definition of environment is that it is the aggregate of surrounding things, conditions, or influences that affect existence and development.

The influence of the nurse on the environment of the elderly varies with the setting. If the elderly person is living in a home, the nurse can assist in positive environmental impact on health and make appropriate suggestions to the person and the family. In an institutional setting, the nurse has more control over the environment. Safety, especially for the elderly person, may require ramps, handrails and other adaptations to accommodate special needs. Comfort measures include provision for privacy; opportunities to function independently when possible; and a psychologically supportive environment with respect for individual differences. The nurse in a nursing home, realizing that the residents have experienced the loss of their previous homes, can do much to enable residents to personalize their present environment and thus maximize their health.

Environment is a crucial element of health. Dunn (1965) defined high level wellness in terms of the relationship between health and environment. Dubos (1965) published extensively in the field of environmental science and health and described health as meaningful only when a person functions in a specific environment. He further challenged society to use the environment to maximize the potential of man.

There are many environmental options for the elderly in the United States. Some live with spouses, siblings, children, friends, and some live alone. They live in housing they have long occupied and neighborhoods they know; in senior high rises where there are others to socialize with; in retirement communities, in rural, urban and suburban locales; in life care communities; and a small percentage live in nursing homes and other institutions.

Powell (1979) has written at length on environmental designs that are supportive to the elderly. In his publication on therapeutic environments for the aged, he stresses the need to consider the availability of emergency services, transportation, security and general concerns for safety that incorporate the sensory losses common in the elderly. Well marked crosswalks, adequate lighting and high intensity auditory signals such as those used in fire alarms and telephones are examples of such adaptations. Powell recommends collaboration between those with knowledge in gerontology and those with knowledge in other areas of planning and design construction that affect the environment of the elderly.

SUMMARY

The promotion and maintenance of health in the aging process is an important arena of action for the gerontological nurse. The federal government has identified health objectives for the nation that seek to promote health and prevent disease in all age groups. Health education is one facet in the implementation of these objectives and nurses provide a major portion of the health education in the health care system.

High level wellness is a concept that identifies a positive direction for health, not just the prevention and treatment of disease. Factors that contribute to this concept are nutrition, physical fitness, stress management, sexuality and environment.

References

Comfort, Alex. *A good age*. New York: Crown Publishers, 1976.

Dubos, R. *Man adapting*. New Haven: Yale University Press, 1965.

Dunn, H. *High level wellness*. Virginia: R.W. Beatty, Ltds, 1961.

Butler, R. and Lewis, M. *Sex after sixty*. New York: Harper & Row Publishers, 1976.

Healthy People. 1979. The Surgeon General's Report on Health Promotion and Disease Prevention. U.S. Dept. of Health, Education and Welfare. Supt. of Documents, U.S. Government Printing Office, Washington, DC. DHEW (PHS) Publication No. 79-55071.

Maslow, Abraham H. *Motivation and personality*. New York: Harper & Row, 1954.

Masters, William H. and Johnson, Virginia E. *Human sexual response*. Boston: Little, Brown, 1966.

McCarthy, P. Geriatric sexuality: Capacity, interest, and opportunity. *Journal of Gerontological Nursing*, 5(1), January-February 1979, 20-24.

Powell, M.L. Therapeutic environments for the aged. In D. Canter and S. Canter (Eds.), *Designing for therapeutic environments*. London: John Wiley, 1979, 233-276.

Promoting health/preventing disease: Objectives for the nation. 1980. U.S. Dept. of Health and Human Services. Supt. of Documents, U.S. Government Printing Office, Washington, DC.

Report on technical committee on health maintenance and health promotion. The 1981 White House Conference on Aging.

SEICUS. *Sexuality and man*. New York: Scribners, 1970.

Selye, J. *The stress of life*. New York: McGraw-Hill Book Co., 1976.

Shine, M.S., Silva, M.C., and Weed, F.S. Integrating health education into baccalaureate nursing curriculum. *Journal of Nursing Education, 22*(1), January 1983, 22-27.

Suggested Readings on Promotion and Maintenance of Health in the Aging Process

Andrews, F.M. and Withey, S.B. *Social indicators of wellbeing: Americans' perception of life quality*. New York: Plenum, 1976.

Archer, S.E., Fleshman, R., Carver, C., and Adelman, L. Lifestyle indicators for interventions to facilitate elderly persons' independence. *Health values: Achieving High Level Wellness. 3*(3), May/June 1979, 129-135.

Butler, R., Gertman, J., Oberlander, D., and Schindler, L. Self-care, self-help, and the elderly. *International Journal of Aging and Human Development*, 1979-80, *10*(1), 95-117.

Cassell, E.J. *The healer's art: A new approach to the doctor-patient relationship*. Philadelphia: Lippincott, 1976.

Cassel, J. The relation of the urban environment to health: Toward a conceptual frame and a research strategy. In L.E. Hinkle, Jr., and W.C. Loring (Eds.), *The effect of the man made environment on health and behavior*. Atlanta: Center for Disease Control, Public Health Service, 1977.

Dubos, R.J. *Man, medicine and environment*. New York: Praeger, 1968.

Gaarder, L. and Cohen, S. *Patient Activated Care for Rural Elderly*. Boise, Idaho: Mountain States Health Corporation. 1982.

Harris, R. and Frankel, L.J. (Eds.). *Guide to Fitness After 50*. New York: Plenum, 1977.

Insel, P.M. and Moos, R.H. (Eds.). *Health and the social environment*. Lexington, MA: Heath, 1974.

Kayser-Jones, J. *Old, Alone and Neglected*. Berkeley: University of California, 1981.

Lazarus, R.S. and Cohen, J.B. Environmental stress. In I. Altman and J.F. Wohlwill (Eds.), *Human behavior and environment*, Vol. 2. New York: Plenum 1977.

Levin, L., Katz, A., and Holst, E. *Self-care: Lay initiatives in health*. New York: Prodist, 1976.

Moos, R. Environmental choice and control in community care settings for older people. *Journal of Applied Social Psychology*, 1981, *11*(1), 23-43.

Noyes, L. Gray and gay. *Journal of Gerontological Nursing*, 1982, *8*(11), 636-639.

Thomas, Ellen G. Application of stress factors in gerontologic nursing. *Nursing Clinics of North America*, December 1979, *14*(4), 607-620.

Yoselle, H. Sexuality in Later Years. In T. Wells (Ed.), *Aging and Health Promotion*. Rockville, MD: Aspen Systems Corp. 1982, 59-72.

4

Health

Deviations

Common to the

Aging Process

Despite improving health status in the growing population of elderly persons in this country, health deviations continue to be a reality. The normal changes in aging contribute to a decline in many functions especially in the seventh and eighth decade of life with chronic illness often compounded by functional disabilities. For the gerontological nurse, this reality requires assessment skills that can differentiate normal aging process from disease, make appropriate referrals and support elderly persons in coping with their illnesses. It is often in old age that people are forced to face chronic illness for the first time. Nurses must be able to assist with adaptation to chronic illness, preferably within a context of existing wellness as described in Chapter III.

In attempting to categorize common health deviations in the elderly, it is apparent that any such attempt is arbitrary. Multiple factors are constantly interacting in the individual in ways that defy categorization. What is physical that does not have psychosocial implications? How can descriptions of mental illness be considered without awareness of physical and social factors that impact on them?

The dilemma has been addressed somewhat conventionally in the following chapter under two general headings of:

1. Physical changes and common health deviations in aging, and
2. Psychosocial and behavioral changes that impede function in aging.

Physical changes encompass the following systems: integumentary, musculoskeletal, endocrine, fluid and electrolyte, sensory, neurological, dental , gastrointestinal, genitourinary, cardiovascular and respiratory. The common psychological and behavioral factors that affect aging are stress, alcoholism, loss, grief, depression and confusion. Drug management is also discussed.

In discussing common changes in aging and diseases that occur, it is recognized that these vary with each individual and are affected by genetic and environmental factors. The information covered in this chapter is based on the current state of the art as it exists in the United States.

PHYSICAL CHANGES AND COMMON HEALTH DEVIATIONS IN AGING

Integumentary System

Because of its visibility, the skin has been seen as a ruthless indicator of age. As with other body changes that occur with aging, skin changes will vary with the individual and may be influenced by genetic characteristics. The expected changes are related to the general thinning of epithelial and subcutaneous fatty layer, changes in fluid balance and endocrine secretions, lifestyle and climate.

Lines and wrinkles, sometimes referred to as furrowing, appear especially on the face. Hair thins on the head and loses its color, while hair on the face in women and in the nose and ears in men increases. Pubic hair is lost in both sexes and men may lose hair on their arms and legs. Brown patches (age spots) are found on the back of the hands, and also on the face, forearms and genitoanal areas. Skin texture becomes rough and mottles in exposed areas especially on light complexioned persons. Nails on the fingers and toes become thick and brittle. Small skin hemorrhages called purpura may be seen on the back of the hands and forearms, and the skin may look paler as blood supply decreases.

Disorders and diseases of the skin are categorized as either infectious or non-infectious (Bruno, 1979). Infectious diseases may be viral, bacterial, fungal or infestations. These infections can be indicative of systemic disease often found in the elderly such as anemia or diabetes.

Non-infectious skin diseases are those due to alterations in cell growth, degenerative changes, hypersensitive reactions, alterations in vascular patterns and positional trauma. Alterations in cell growth produce tumors that may be benign, pre-malignant or malignant. Cancer of the skin is a common malignancy in elderly persons. Degenerative changes are reflected in hyperkeratosis such as that seen in calluses and corns. Hypersensitive reactions include immune reactions.

TABLE 4-1
Changes in the integumentary system in old age

Normal changes	Abnormal changes
Thinning of epithelial cells and subcutaneous fat layers	Infections - viral
Lines and wrinkles in skin	bacterial
Thinning and loss of color in hair	fungal
Age spots	Abnormal cell growth and tumors
Roughness and dryness in skin	benign
Thickening and brittleness in nails	malignant
	Skin ulcerations

Nursing implications. The nurse is often the person who has the most opportunity to observe the skin of elderly persons who are receiving nursing care. In addition to distinguishing normal from abnormal changes, the nurse can assist the person in managing their own health by providing information on these changes and how to respond to them. Minimizing sun exposure by shade or use of sun screeners, and keeping the skin moisturized are important in preventing skin damage. Frequent turning and care of pressure areas is a prime nursing responsibility for persons who are bedridden or otherwise unable to move themselves freely. Examination of the skin regularly by the person or primary caretaker for changes in pigmentation or lumps is essential. Appropriate referrals to dermatologists can be initiated and facilitated by the nurse.

Alterations in vascular patterns contribute to the common condition of osteosis in which the skin is very dry, itchy and less effective as a barrier against infection. Positional trauma is seen in skin ulcerations on tissue over boney prominences such as the common decubitus ulcer on the lower back of persons who are bedridden.

Protection of the skin from sun and trauma and moistening of dry skin are important elements of general care of the elderly. Skin permeability decreases with age, making the use of ointments less effective.

Musculoskeletal System

Growing old is often associated with expected rheumatism and arthritis. Fractures, especially prior to modern treatment, terrified the elderly because they were often associated with dire consequences due to prolonged immobility and resultant pneumonia, skin breakdown and other complications. Current medical practice has eliminated many of the hazards of prolonged convalescence following fractures, although hip fractures continue to cause justifiable alarm. The factor most responsible for increased susceptibility to fractures is osteoporosis, a common metabolic disease especially in white elderly women, that decreases the quantity of bone thus weakening its density and structure. These bone changes also contribute to the loss of height that is common in older persons due to changes in the spine. Increased calcium intake and regular exercising are important in the prevention and treatment of bone problems caused by osteoporosis.

In addition to bone changes, there are changes in the joints and muscles that occur with aging. Cartilage deteriorates and there may be boney growths at the edge of joints. According to Shanck (1981), age is a predisposing factor in primary osteoarthritis, a disease that affects forty million people. This is a non-inflammatory condition found in movable joints and it especially affects the weight-bearing joints such as the hips and knees as well as the spine. This disease is responsible for much pain and immobility in the elderly population. Conservative treatment generally consists of heat application and exercise to the affected joint.

A second form of arthritis—rheumatoid arthritis—is a systemic disease that is inflammatory and affects connective tissues in the joints. In this disease, there is inflammation of the synovial membrane with accompanying swelling, heat and tenderness. This disease is chronic and progressive although it does have periods of remissions and exacerbations. Disability and deformity result from this disease. Medical treatment for rheumatoid arthritis is mainly focused on reducing inflammation with aspirin or other anti-inflammatory medicines. Other drugs and metals, such as gold, are sometimes prescribed.

Surgery is performed when needed in the treatment of arthritis. Psy-

TABLE 4-2
Changes in the musculoskeletal system in old age

Normal changes	Abnormal changes
Loss of flexibility in joints	Osteoporosis
Cartilage degeneration	Arthritis
Boney growths at edge of joints	osteoarthritis
	rheumatoid arthritis
	Fractures
	Loss of height due to spinal
	column changes

chological support to the person having pain and disability due to arthritis is an important aspect of nursing care and is combined with the health measures described in Chapter III.

In addition to the common diseases mentioned, some of the common changes in the musculoskeletal system that occur in aging include kyphosis, muscle weakness and flabbiness in the arms, legs and hips, muscle tremors and cramping, decrease in abdominal reflexes and enlarged joints.

Nursing implications. The nurse can assist the elderly person in adjusting to the normal aging changes in the musculoskeletal system by supplying information on ways to minimize the effects of these changes. The need for regular exercise, both stretching and strengthening, can be stressed, and available classes for these exercises in the community can be publicized, including those on television. Dietary supplements such as calcium for women with osteoporosis is suggested by many doctors. For persons who are limited in mobility, environmental supports to enable them to function within their limits can be provided in institutions and recommended to family caretakers in the home. Pain management and comfort are nursing considerations for the many elderly persons with arthritis and related diseases.

Endocrine System

Aging changes affect the endocrine system primarily by decreases in hormones secreted and changes in the endocrine glands. Thyroid activity and basal metabolism rate slow down. Adrenal glands decrease in function and this further affects the thyroid function and decreases the capacity to handle stress. The pituitary gland becomes smaller in weight. These and other hormonal changes contribute to a variety of functional changes that vary from one individual to another.

The most common endocrine related disease that occurs with increasing frequency with age is diabetes mellitus. This disease results from abnormal secretions of the pancreas, especially insulin, which disturb the regular metabolism of carbohydrates, fats and proteins. The four major results of the disturbance are: hyperglycemia, large blood vessel disease such as atherosclerosis and arteriosclerosis; microvascular disease which is frequently evidenced in the kidney and the eye; and peripheral neuropathy which usually involves sensory nerves in the lower extremities (Blainey, 1979). This disease often causes symptoms of decreased motility in the gastrointestinal and urinary systems and is sometimes associated with sexual impotence. The treatment of diabetes requires detailed information and ongoing support to the elderly person and the family. Diet management, insulin administration and the control of activity and stress are important factors.

TABLE 4-3
Changes in the endocrine system in old age

Normal changes	Abnormal changes
Decrease in hormones	Diabetes
Decrease in basal metabolism	Hypothyroidism
Decrease in gland function	Hyperthyroidism
Decrease in size of pituitary gland	

Nursing implications. It is important that the nurse recognize the general slowing down of function in the endocrine system and its impact on the metabolism of foods and drugs. In caring for elderly persons with diabetes, diet management, insulin administration, activity and stress control are important and teaching programs for patients and families who are managing diabetes are available in many hospitals and clinics. These same factors are important in the treatment and management of other diseases related to the endocrine system. Since endocrine disease is not always as readily diagnosed or as clear in its symptoms as diseases in systems that have visible external manifestations, the nurse can help by being empathic with persons who are frustrated by the vagueness of symptoms and the difficulty in medical diagnosis. Support to the person and the family in dealing with symptoms and managing the environment is crucial.

Fluid and Electrolyte Balance

In the aged person, there is a decline in the total body water due to a shift in the fluid balance. Intracellular fluid decreases while extracellular fluid remains the same. A common problem seen in the elderly due to fluid and electrolyte imbalance is dehydration. Edema may also result. Imbalances in fluid and electrolytes contribute to acidosis or alkalosis, conditions that require careful monitoring when being treated in the elderly. Decreased functioning of the liver and kidneys affects the body's ability to maintain electrolyte balance, and the overall regulatory mechanisms of the body may be less able to adapt to imbalance. In replacing fluids it is important to watch for pulmonary edema caused by overload that cannot be handled in a fragile cardiovascular system.

The nurse in an institutional setting needs to monitor fluid intake and output on patients with fluid and electrolyte imbalance. The nurse in the clinic or home care setting needs to instruct the person or caretaker on this type of monitoring.

Sensory Losses in Aging

Sensory losses that occur with aging interfere with the individuals ability to see, hear, taste, smell and touch. Although most of these losses develop gradually, they represent a major fear in the elderly. The following is a summary of common changes in sensory organs and capacity that are associated with age.

Sight: In the aging process, normal vision changes occur that affect sight, including presbyopia. Acuity is decreased, accommodation is altered, adaptation to light and darkness slows down, and there may be increased difficulty in discriminating between colors. The most common diseases that affect sight are cataracts, glaucoma and senile macular degeneration.

Cataracts are the most common visual disorder in the United States and two thirds of the cataract surgery performed is on older adults. The National Eye Institute defines a cataract as a cloudiness or opacity in the lens of the eye which interferes with vision. It is not a tumor or a film over the eye and can be surgically treated whenever it interferes seriously with sight rather than waiting for total blindness or "ripeness" as was sometimes done in the past. Surgery is usually successful in treating this condition and new types of surgery such as microsurgery and laser treatment have lessened the time needed to recover. Contact lenses are often used after surgery although many patients continue to wear cataract glasses.

A second disease process that interferes with sight is glaucoma which is the third leading cause of blindness in the United States. Glaucoma represents a group of eye diseases. It is recognized by increased pressure of fluid within the eye, changes in the optic disk and losses in the visual field. The disease occurs in two percent of middle-aged adults and the occurrence increases to ten percent by the eighth and ninth decades of life. Treatment of glaucoma is medical and is usually accomplished with drugs in the form of eye drops instilled regularly. Once glaucoma is diagnosed, it is considered a lifetime condition and, like diabetes, requires lifetime treatment and management. This type of non-reversible diagnosis may contribute to depression or other symptoms of adaptation problems in some people and they need to be given support in handling their loss and incorporating treatment into their lifestyle.

Senile macular degeneration (SMD) is a third disease that interferes with sight. A National Eye Institute study in 1979 showed that the incidence of

TABLE 4-4
Sensory changes in old age

Normal changes	Abnormal changes
Sight	
Presbyopia	Cataracts
Lowered acuity	Glaucoma
Altered accommodation to light and dark	Senile macular degeneration
Difficulty in color discrimination	
Hearing	
Presbycusis	Deafness
Excessive wax (cerumen)	
Touching	
Lowering of ability to distinguish hot and cold and feel pain	Total loss of feeling
Taste	
Lowered ability to distinguish specific tastes	Total loss of taste
Smell	
Lowered ability to distinguish specific odors	Total loss of smell

SMD is 1.6% in the 52-64 age group, 11% in the 65-74 age group and 27.9% in the 75-84 age group. The macula, which is the location in the retina where there is greatest visual acuity, loses its function possibly due to lowered blood supply to nerve endings in that area. The disease usually affects both eyes and is characterized by interference in straightforward vision. Signs and symptoms differ in individuals making diagnosis difficult. Peripheral vision is not affected initially and is often used as a substitute by persons with SMD. Laser therapy is currently considered the best available treatment.

Hearing: The aging process is often accompanied by unilateral or bilateral hearing loss. Presbycusis is the name given to progressive hearing loss due to age. This generally affects the inner ear and the retrocochlea, with high frequency sounds among the first to be lost. Some forms of deafness are treatable with hearing aids, and surgery is a consideration for specific hearing defects. Differential diagnoses are crucial and the elderly person needs referral to an audiologist to assist in distinguishing causes of deafness. For the elderly person who is not able to compensate for or cure deafness, environmental adjustments are needed. Carty (1972) has described some of the special needs of deaf people as these relate to nursing care.

Taste: Elderly persons can experience a significant loss of taste sensation. The ability to distinguish sweet and salty tastes is the first to decline. The major consequence of taste loss is in its influence on the desire for nutritious food.

Smell: The sense of smell is closely associated with taste. This sense also lessens with age and affects the elderly person's ability to distinguish odors. One of the major problems associated with the loss of smell, in additon to lessening the ability to smell food, is the inability to notice offensive body odors. While this may be a blessing to the person who is unable to smell, by ignoring personal odors that offend others the elderly person can inadvertently put himself in a position of social isolation.

Touch: Age affects the ability to feel and lessens the person's ability to distinguish hot and cold and to feel pain. The consequences of these losses have obvious safety implications since pain warns us of problems and extremes of heat and cold can cause damage. In addition to these obvious outcomes of tactile loss, there is the more primal expression of touch that allows us to feel objects and persons as a way of understanding what they are and of communicating with those that are alive.

Elderly persons experiencing problems due to sensory loss need to seek diagnostic help and treatment as soon as possible to allow early intervention and correction of problems when possible.

Nursing implications. The nurse who recognizes sensory losses in elderly persons can assist in providing an environment that will minimize the functional effects of these losses. Providing sufficient light can help with sight difficulty and use of large print in material to be read and in medication labelling is important. For those who have difficulty hearing, minimizing background noises during conversation, and speaking slowly and directly to the person help. Correct glasses and hearing aids when appropriate provide relief from these losses and the nurse can be the person to provide referrals. The use of dogs to assist persons with sight and hearing losses is increasing and voluntary as well as official community agencies exist to help with blindness and deafness in persons of all ages, including the aged.

Losses in taste and smell affect appetite and may result in nutritional deficiency. Nurses can encourage that meals be prepared that are more attractive to the individual. In caring for an elderly person who has significantly diminished sense of touch, the nurse will need to take extra steps to assure that the person receives sensory stimulation in taking the person's hand with both of the nurse's hands and taking the time to allow the person to feel the personal contact despite lowered sensory perception. In carrying out nursing procedures, it is important to remember that heat and cold response may be damaged and the nurse may need to watch for signs of extremes that can be harmful if the patient is unable to distinguish these.

Neurological System

The neurological system, which encompasses the brain as well as the central, peripheral and autonomic nervous systems, changes physically with age. The postmitotic nerve cells are not replaced when they die and this results in a loss of brain weight and of parts of the cerebral cortex. There is an increase in fatty substances called senile plaques that are seen as interfering with mental functioning (Goldman, 1979). Reduction in the cerebral blood flow and the decreasing metabolism in the aged are seen as contributing to loss of intellectual functioning. Nerve conduction velocity changes and this decreases response time and interferes with perception. Sensory perception is decreased and sleep patterns change.

Common disease processes of the neurological system in the aged are cerebrovascular diseases, Parkinson's disease, and Alzheimer's disease and related disorders.

The most commonly recognized outcome of cerebrovascular disease is the "cerebrovascular accident" (CVA) also called a stroke. The three main causes of stroke are: a) cerebral thrombosis, b) cerebral embolism, and c) cerebral hemorrhage. Atherosclerosis and hypertension increase the risk of a stroke occurring.

Strokes occur with increasing frequency after the age of sixty, are twice as common in men as in women and result in death for 40 percent of their victims. Of the persons who live after a stroke, according to the National Institute of Neurological and Communicative Disorders and Strokes, 30 percent return to work and normal life activity; 55 percent are disabled but with assistance can carry on the activities of daily living; and 15 percent are totally dependent on others for their care.

A transient ischemic attack (TIA), sometimes called a "little stroke", result when there is a temporary lack of blood to a part of the brain. These are reversible, but they often precede a major stroke and can serve as a warning of a high risk for stroke.

Consequences of a stroke depend on the location. Paralysis on one or both sides, visual and sensory loss, incontinence, and speech defects are the most common consequences, with motor and sensory loss contributing to rehabilitation complications. Treatment of stroke is usually medical with emphasis on controlling the cause, minimizing the chance of recurrence and supporting maximum rehabilitation. Occasionally surgical treatment is used to remove clots. Rehabilitation of the elderly person who has suffered a stroke is a major challenge to gerontological nurses.

Parkinson's disease is a degenerative neurological disease which progresses slowly and often leads to severe disability and dependence. It is characterized by tremors, rigidity in muscles and slowness of motor activity. A person with Parkinson's disease has difficulty controlling body movements due to the disease processes in the central nervous system which are often associated with cerebral vascular disease and arteriosclerosis in aging. Medications are used to control symptoms while exercise and massage can be used to increase joint mobility and give some comfort.

Alzheimer's disease and related disorders are responsible for what has historically been called "senile dementia" or "senility", the dreaded disease that impairs the intellectual functioning of 3 to 4 million elderly Americans. (Progress Report on Senile Dementia of the Alzheimer's Type, 1981). Alzheimer's disease can occur as early as 40 years of age and there is scientific controversy over whether the disease is the same as senile dementia or different. Current terminology for the disease when it occurs in persons over the age of 65 is senile dementia of the Alzheimer's type (SDAT), and it is estimated that 500,000 elderly Americans have this type of senile dementia.

The common changes seen in SDAT are in the proteins of the nerve cells and lead to an accumulation of neurofibrillary tangles. Different patterns and rates of deterioration in both mental and neurological functioning occur in SDAT. Common symptoms include increased memory loss, confusion, irritability, agitation and personality changes.

Other conditions that produce similar symptoms are vascular disorders such as strokes, brain tumors, drug reactions, thyroid dysfunction, and infectious and pernicious anemia. It is important to distinguish the cause of severe intellectual impairment in the elderly. Some of the causes can be corrected and the process of the resultant dementia can be reversed. The progress of SDAT is not reversible at the present time and since its etiology is unknown, its treatment is mainly symptomatic.

Federal funds for research on SDAT have increased markedly during the past five years. The National Institute on Aging, the National Institute of Neurological and Communicative Disorders and Stroke, and the National Institute of Mental Health have all collaborated in seeking new research on SDAT. A national voluntary health association called the Alzheimer's Disease and Related Disorders Association has been formed by families of victims of Alzheimer's disease to increase public awareness of this problem and to suppport self-help groups.

TABLE 4-5
Changes in the neurological system in old age

Normal Changes	Abnormal Changes
General slowing down of reaction time	Cerebrovascular disease
Slow response to heat and cold	Parkinson's disease
Changing sleep patterns	Senile dementia including Alzheimer's
Decreased cerebral blood flow	disease

Nursing implications. One of the most difficult consequences of neurological disease is the change in personality of the individual and the resultant loss of desired responses and communication. This type of change affects all who are in contact with the individual, especially those responsible for care of dependent elderly persons. The possibility of a burnout syndrome in health care providers is a professional concern and needs attention in institutions that provide long-term care to elderly persons with dementia. This hazard also occurs with family members who are providing full time care at home. Nurses who are working with these families need to recognize the need for support systems and refer families to community resources such as day care, respite care and personal counselling and support groups.

Dental Changes with Aging

Dental changes with aging often result in loss of teeth. This is usually due to inflammatory bone resorption around teeth, a form of osteoporosis. The resorption of the gum tissue near the base of teeth exposes more of the teeth and gives an elongated appearance. Surfaces of the teeth also wear down with wear and tooth enamel may be lost. Dental caries are seen in the elderly, often at the base of the teeth.

Correct fitting dentures are crucial to the dental health of those who have lost teeth. Regular dental checkups are strongly advised for the elderly to increase the chance of early interventions that can eliminate the need for losing teeth. A suggestion that the nurse can make to assist in removing plaque from teeth is that after bathing, people can wipe their teeth with the towel used to dry their bodies. This stimulates gum circulation in addition to removing plaque and doing this at bath times makes it easier to remember.

TABLE 4-6
Dental changes in old age

Normal Changes	Abnormal Changes
Surfaces of teeth wear down	Gum disease
Gum tissue recedes	Caries

Nursing implications. For the dependent elderly person, mouth care is fundamental to good nursing care. In addition to keeping the mouth clean, moistening with water-soluble lubricants will prevent excessive dryness due to open mouth breathing or medications that cause dryness. Elderly persons who are taking care of their own dental needs can be encouraged to check regularly with their dentist or dental hygienist for removal of plaque and identification of caries, especially those that develop along the gumline. For the person wearing dentures, correct fit and cleanliness are important.

Gastrointestinal System

The gastrointestinal system is vulnerable to a number of age-related changes and diseases that interfere with ingestion, digestion and elimination. Some of these changes are anatomical and some are physiological. They affect both the structure and the function of this system causing anxiety in the older person and frustration in those assuming responsibility of care.

Common anatomical changes occur in the esophagus which dilates and empties more slowly, in the diaphragm region with hiatal hernias that allow the stomach to ease up into the chest cavity through weaknesses in the diaphragm wall, decreased muscle tone in the small and large intestines, diverticulosis especially in the sigmoid colon and loss of tone in the rectal sphincter muscles.

Concurrent with these structural changes, there is a general slowing down of motility and peristalsis in the intestinal tract, a decrease in the production of digestive enzymes, a decrease in absorption and utilization of essential minerals and nutrients and an increase in diseases. As in all system changes, it is important to remember that the rate and intensity of change due to aging is individual and that, even within different systems in the same individual, there will be different rates of change with resultant differences in pathology and disease.

Common disorders include those found in the various structures within the gastrointestinal system and those that are systemic in origin but impact on the digestive system.

Hiatal hernias occur in forty to sixty percent of the elderly (Bartol and Heitkemper, 1979). Although most of these are without persistent symptoms, they may cause heartburn, pain and pressure in the xiphoid region. Pain from this condition and from esophageal distress must be differentiated from cardiac symptoms and occur in the same region.

In the stomach, there is an increase in gastritis. Abbey (1981) has categorized three types of gastritis found in the elderly: acute, chronic hypertrophic and chronic atrophic. Acute gastritis is caused by specific agents such as bacterial toxins from food, or drugs, is self-limiting when the agent is removed, and is treated with antacids and general health measures. Chronic hypertrophic gastritis causes burning pain and dyspepsia due to inflammed rugae. Chronic atrophic gastritis varies in severity and is caused by mucosal atrophy and decreased function of gastric glands with resultant decrease in the production of hydrochloric acid. Pernicious anemia may result from decreased absorption of vitamin B_{12} in this condition.

Ulcers occur with increasing frequency with age. These may be gastric or peptic and their complications when they are bleeding are serious and even fatal in the elderly. Medical treatment is preferred, with surgery used only when medical treatment is not effective.

Common problems in the intestines are obstructions, diverticulosis and problems in absorption. Absorption problems are associated with the changes of aging that influence enzyme production, digestive motility and changes in structure. Obstruction may be due to paralysis of the intestine or due to a mechanical cause such as a tumor. Diverticulosis is a herniation of the colon

TABLE 4-7
Gastrointestinal changes in old age

Normal	Abnormal
Decrease in rate of motility in peristalsis	Constipation
Decrease in pancreatic function	Diarrhea
Esophagus empties and dilates more slowly	Gastritis
Decrease in gastric acid	Hiatal hernia
Increase in flatus	Fecal incontinence
	Gallstones
	Intestinal obstruction
	Diverticulitis
	Cancer

mucosa through the muscle and is most common in the sigmoid area.

Changes in the liver, gallbladder and pancreas impact on the digestive system. The liver decreases in size with age. The pancreas decreases in function but increases in fat. Biliary stones increase in the gallbladder with gallstones found in twenty percent of the elderly.

Problems with elimination increase with age and are on a continuum that runs from fecal impaction and constipation to fecal incontinence and diarrhea with the desired function being normalcy as it was experienced by the individual during his earlier life.

Fecal impaction sometimes occurs in individuals with chronic constipation and low levels of activity. Treatment consists of manual removal of the impaction and measures to prevent its recurrence.

Constipation is a condition frequently talked about among the elderly, advertised on the media and often perceived as normal. It is estimated that one fourth of the population over sixty take laxatives regularly. Bartol and Heitkemper (1979) describe three forms of constipation: hypertonic, hypotonic and habit. Constipation that is due to habits of diet lacking in bulk or due to ignoring the urge to defecate consistently can be treated with modification of behaviors. Constipation due to toning losses in the bowel can be treated with laxatives, enemas, and suppositories. Drugs that contribute to constipation should be assessed for their effects, and neurological diseases that affect colon function need to be considered in treating this problem.

Diarrhea and fecal incontinence create problems of skin care for the elderly person and those caring for him. It is estimated that twenty percent of hospitalized elderly patients have fecal incontinence, some of this due to confusion and/or neurologic changes. Diarrhea affects the elderly more seriously than the younger population due to the danger of potassium and sodium imbalance and saline depletion. The treatment of diarrhea depends on assessing the cause; this condition is a potential medical emergency in the elderly.

Cancer in the gastrointestinal system is a serious problem for the elderly. Cancer of the colon and rectum occurs most often in elderly persons (Molbo, 1979). Cancer of the esophagus increases with age. Treatment of cancer in the elderly is similar to other age groups with the necessity to evaluate its consequences based on the changes of aging and the resultant adaptations needed.

Nursing implications. In addition to nursing measures for specific diseases of the gastrointestinal system the nurse can initiate, or encourage the elderly person or family to initiate, eating habits that will help the function of the aging digestive tract. Increased fluid intake plus use of bulk in the diet such as bran, can promote healthy patterns of elimination. Persons may need information on what is normal in bowel function – this is usually determined by past history. Remaining upright after meals will ease discomfort from slow digestion. In monitoring drug use in elderly persons, it is important that the nurse consider the reduced activity in the digestive tract and allow for clearance in this tract and in the liver before administering further doses of medications.

Genitourinary System

There are obvious differences in the genitourinary systems of men and women and there are equally obvious commonalities related to aging changes. There is a tendency for muscles to lose their elasticity and for supportive structures to lose their tone. Kidney functional units decline with resultant decline in overall kidney function. This is not in itself a serious problem since kidneys can support body functions with fifty percent function. It becomes a problem when disease processes place extra demands on kidney functioning and when medications are used.

Frequency and urgency increase with age due to some of the changes mentioned above and need to be managed so as not to interfere with activities. Urinary incontinence is a condition dreaded by both the elderly and their caretakers and is often used as the criteria for capability of independent living style vs. custodial care. Field (1979), has categorized two types of urinary incontinence: 1) spurious or related to environmental factors, and 2) central or related to physiologic factors. Environmental factors include difficulty in getting to a toilet in time and increased fluid intake at bedtime. Physiologic causes of incontinence include disorders of neurological control, urethra, bladder, pelvic diaphragm and unstable bladders. Treatment for urinary incontinence at this time varies and may include physiotherapy, electrical stimulation and behavior therapy for retraining. Surgery is somtimes done when indicated but must be carefully evaluated in an aged person.

Urinary tract infection (UTI) risk increases with age especially in men who have prostatic obstruction and women who have cystoceles. Usual signs of infection such as fever, confusion and illness are accompanied by specific symptoms of frequency, urgency, dysuria, lower abdominal discomfort and possibly hematuria. Some elderly persons with UTI do not report these symptoms or do not seem to have them despite existing UTI. Treatment of this problem is primarily done with antimicrobial drugs and increased fluid intake. Women are sometimes treated preventively with estrogen cream.

Prostatic obstruction due to enlargement of the prostate gland occurs in thirty percent of males over fifty years of age. The enlargement or hypertrophy of the prostate may be benign or malignant. Cancer of the prostate is the third most common male malignancy and is the most common site for tumors in males over eighty years of age. The progress of cancer in the elderly is slower than in younger age groups and treatment considerations weigh the side effects of surgery, radiation and chemotherapy against life expectancy. If symptoms of the disease are not expected to interfere with functions during a lifetime, some persons choose not to accept active treatment.

In elderly women, a common genitourinary problem is atrophic vaginitis. Estrogen depletion with age results in a vulnerability to trauma and infection in the vagina due to the lack of secretions to the epithelium cells. Symptoms include soreness and itching in the vagina and vulva with pain during sexual intercourse and often a continuous thin discharge. Perineal hygiene to assure cleanliness can minimize the possibility of secondary infections. Estrogen replacement, either locally with ointments or systemically, is sometimes given. Other vaginal infections such as candida and trichomoniasis may occur in the elderly although these are more common in younger populations.

In working with elderly women and men who have problems that involve sexual organs, caregivers need to be sensitive to their individual attitudes and needs toward sex. This topic is covered in more detail in Chapter III.

TABLE 4-8
Genitourinary changes in old age

Normal	Abnormal
Decreased muscle tone in supportive structures	Prostatic obstruction
	Urinary tract infections
Normal sexual changes	Vaginal infections
Bladder diverticulitis	Vaginitis
Decreased bladder capacity	Urinary incontinence
Prostatic enlargement	Cancer / tumors

Nursing implications. Information to elderly persons and their caretakers about what is normal for the genitourinary system can be given by the nurse to assist in distinguishing disease processes from normal age-related changes. Monitoring of the relationship between fluid intake and output can provide a basis for expected functional level. Environmental support for managing difficulties, such as ready access to a toilet or commode, can help to maintain acceptable function. The nurse needs to be aware of the possibility of infection as a cause of incontinence and refer to the physician for appropriate tests.

Cardiovascular System

Cardiovascular disease is responsible for over half of the deaths in the aged population. Forty percent of those over age sixty-five die of cardiovascular disease; another fifteen percent die of cerebrovascular disease (Goldman, 1979). There are both physical and physiologic changes in the cardiovascular system that contribute to health deviations. Physical changes include increase in the size of the heart, increased collagen, thickening and rigidity of the valves and blood vessels. Physiologically there is a decrease in cardiac output with subsequent decrease in supply of blood to organs, a decrease in cardiac reserve and an increase in vascular resistance. The decrease in blood flow to organs is not symmetrical and more blood continues to flow to the brain and coronary vessels in proportion to other organs such as the kidneys which receive proportionately less flow.

Roberts (1981) has identified two major cardiovascular diseases that increase with age: a) hypertension and b) coronary artery disease. She identifies hypertension as present when the blood pressure is consistently over 170/95 after several visits to record this. Eliopoulos (1979) describes 200/100 as the diagnostic basis for hypertension in the elderly. There continues to be controversy regarding what level of blood pressure is "normal" in the elderly. There is also support for the concept that rather than an absolute figure, diagnosis should be based on comparative data for an individual over a period of time.

Whatever the blood pressure reading, other symptoms such as dull morning headaches, memory impairment, confusion and disorientation usually send the client to the physician, and medication, dietary and lifestyle management measures are prescribed to alleviate symptoms and lower blood pressure. For persons who are asymptomatic in the presence of high blood pressure, the need for preventive measures must be explained. In some instances, signs and symptoms of low blood pressure such as fatigue and dizziness send elderly people for care. It is important to monitor low blood pressure and look for causes.

Coronary artery disease occurs when the collateral circulation which develops after normal atherosclerosis of the coronary arteries is insufficient to meet circulation needs. The most common symptom for this disease is angina which may vary from mild to severe. Elderly persons may report less pain from angina and even from acute coronary occlusion than younger persons but they often have more dyspnea.

Congestive heart failure is a common complication of coronary artery disease and reflects a decompensation of the heart pumping function in a person with heart disease. Characteristic symptoms are edema, dyspnea on exertion, coughing, oliguria, confusion and chronic fatigue (Atwood, 1979). Treatment for congestive heart disease is mainly focused on changes in lifestyle such as low sodium diet and adjustment of exertion to balance with cardiac capacity. Diuretics may also be used.

In addition to the occurrence of diseases specific to the heart, the aged have an increased occurrence of peripheral vascular disease especially in the lower extremities. These are often categorized as either acute or chronic. Acute obstructive disease results when emboli or thrombi suddenly obstruct the blood vessel. This results in cutting off circulation with accompanying symptoms of pain, color changes and cyanosis and can continue on to gangrene. The blood clot is often removed surgically and amputation is seen as a last resort.

Chronic obstructive vascular disease is a gradual process with resultant ischemia from the reduction in blood vessel function. Treatment is generally conservative and aims at reducing risk factors such as obesity and smoking, and adjusting activity and rest to maximize circulation and minimize pain.

Another common occurrence in the elderly vascular system is the presence of varicose veins. These are especially apt to be found in persons with a family history of this problem, in those who stand frequently in their work and in women who have had many pregnancies. The condition is a dilation of the superficial leg veins and these are seen as enlarged veins on the leg with accompanying pain, discoloration and leg fatigue. Surgical intervention by stripping/ligating the veins, and injection of hypertonic fluid to shrink them are used.

TABLE 4-9
Cardiovascular changes in old age

Normal	Abnormal
Increase in size of heart	Hypertension
Increase in collagen	Coronary artery disease
Increase in thickness of valves and	Congestive heart disease
blood vessels	Peripheral vascular disease
Decrease in cardiac output	Varicose veins
Decrease in cardiac reserve	
Decrease in blood flow to organs	

Nursing implications. Prevention is an important factor in alleviating the symptoms of cardiac and vascular disease. Proper diet, exercise, stress management and regular checkups for hidden symptoms such as high blood pressure can be encouraged by the nurse. For the nurse who is giving direct care to elderly persons, observation of signs that normal aging function is becoming pathological can result in early treatment of disease conditions. For persons with circulatory problems in their legs, support hose and frequent elevation of the affected leg can be helpful.

Respiratory System

Physiological changes in the respiratory system that occur in aging include increased anterior/posterior diameter of the chest, progressive kyphosis sometimes complicated by osteoporosis, calcification of costal cartilages, lowered rib mobility, and partial contraction of the muscles of inspiration. Cartilage connecting the ribs to the spinal column and sternum calcifies as does the cartilage in the trachea and bronchi; ciliary processes decrease with progressive atrophy of epithelial cells in the trachea and bronchi; and viscous mucus production is increased due to degeneration of the glands of the respiratory tubules (Rockstein and Sussman, 1979). The elastin content of the lungs increases although the collagen remains the same. There is a decrease in the vital capacity although the total lung capacity remains unchanged. With less air inhaled, there is less oxygen available and thus the older person has less energy. There is also a decrease in coughing ability that interferes with getting rid of excess mucus.

Common respiratory diseases in the elderly are asthma, bronchitis, emphysema, pneumonia and tuberculosis. Chronic obstructive pulmonary disease (COPD) is seen as a combination of chronic bronchitis, asthma and emphysema with persistent obstruction to bronchial air flow and resultant ventilation-perfusion abnormalities in the lungs (Bither, 1979). Breathing becomes more difficult in all of these diseases with the increase in secretions, and energy to maintain activities of daily living becomes scarce. These are considered chronic diseases and require long-term management and appropriate lifestyle adjustments. Respiratory health is enhanced by avoiding smoking and air pollution and by learning good breathing habits.

Signs and symptoms of COPD include coughing, shortness of breath, wheezing, sputum expectorating and changes in pulmonary function studies. These diseases are treated with drugs (bronchodilators, antibiotics), oxygen, fluids, humidification, restricted activities as needed, breathing exercises and postural drainage.

Pneumonia occurs more frequently in the elderly than in younger age groups and is the fourth highest cause of death in those over age seventy-five. This is an acute infectious disease characterized by inflammation of the lungs and occurs more frequently in the winter and spring seasons. Pneumonia brings sudden chills, fever, increased pulse and respiration, and chest pain. In elderly persons, confusion and weakness may be early signs of pneumonia. It is diagnosed by blood test (for leucocytosis) and x-ray. Treatment usually includes rest, antibiotics, oxygen if needed, fluids and careful monitoring for signs of complications.

Tuberculosis is a communicable disease with a peak incidence in the older age groups. Occurrence is usually a reinfection of an earlier episode. Activation of tuberculosis requires a report to public health agencies who provide treatment and education in the care and control of the disease. Current drugs render this disease noncommunicable in shorter periods of time than in the past. Isolation techniques can be used if needed and improvement of general health is recommended for recovery.

The pharynx and larynx are considered part of the respiratory system and, like many other muscles, these atrophy with age. This may result in a lessening of voice power in the elderly and more energy may be needed to talk and be heard, especially in persons with Parkinson's disease.

TABLE 4-10
Respiratory changes in old age

Normal	Abnormal
Increase in the anterior/posterior diameter of the chest	Asthma
Decrease in coughing ability	Bronchitis
Decrease in vital capacity	Emphysema
Increase in mucus production	Pneumonia
Progressive kyphosis	Tuberculosis
Calcification of cartilage connecting ribs to spinal column and sternum	

Nursing implications. The nurse can encourage exercise to improve lung capacity. Increased fluid intake is helpful for respiratory function and environmental support such as the use of a humidifier in heating systems will lessen irritation due to dry air inhalation.

PSYCHOSOCIAL CHANGES THAT IMPEDE FUNCTIONS IN AGING

In addition to the physical changes and diseases that represent health deviations in the elderly, there are psychosocial changes and diseases that interfere with health. Butler and Lewis (1982) describe common emotional problems in the elderly as those related to loss and to reactions to age-related crises including retirement, changing marital and sexual relationships, decreased income, disease, pain, dying and death. They further describe functional disorders such as schizophrenic and paranoid disorders, neuroses and disorders related to affect, anxiety, dissociation and personality.

Eliopoulos (1979) has listed the five most common mental health problems in the elderly as depression, organic brain syndrome, anxiety, paranoia and hypochondriasis. Some of the factors contributing to these and to lowered psychosocial function will be further described.

Stress

Stress activates a more serious response in the elderly than in younger persons due to decreased ability to adapt quickly and compensate for stress reactions.

Burnside (1981) has identified three of the factors that most effect stress: lack of social bonds, suddenness of events, and lack of control over events.

Elderly persons are more likely to react to stress than younger age groups. One stress response is loss of memory. This is usually temporary, but if the stress response is serious, the memory may be permanently damaged. The death of a spouse and a final move into new housing are seen as the two most stressful events for elderly persons. In a study by Wolanin (1981) mortality rates were increased in direct association with preparation for final moves.

Eliopoulos (1979) includes physiological changes such as lowered energy, changing body image and physical limitations as causes of stress in the elderly. Social changes such as retirement, loss of income, and death of family members and friends also produce stress. The attitudes of those whom the elderly person respects such as friends and society impact on the self concept of the individuals. These attitudes are also reflected in the social policies and support systems that are supported in society.

Alcoholism

According to a special report by the U.S. Public Health Service on Alcohol and the Elderly (1982), approximately ten percent of the elderly population has some form of alcohol related problem. The decreased tolerance for alcohol due to the slowing down of metabolism and the increased sensitivity of the nervous system in the elderly contribute to the problem when it exists. Elderly widowers and persons experiencing stress and/or major lifestyle changes and those who are bored or depressed are especially at risk for alcoholism.

Loss

A predominant theme in aging is loss and the elderly have survived more losses than most younger people by reason of longevity. Preston (1979) has divided loss in the elderly into two major categories: interpersonal and intrapersonal. Interpersonal loss is manifested in loneliness which is seen as a personal suffering that is associated with the need or desire for intimacy that is not being fulfilled. This represents losses of people who were cherished, lifestyle, transportation potential, locations, money, health and roles. This type of loneliness is more severe at times that had previously been spent with persons and in places that were lost, such as holidays, evenings, and weekends. This type of loss is best managed by activities and relationships that can compensate for those that are no longer available.

Intrapersonal loss in the elderly is characterized not only by the loss of cherished relationships, attributes and material possessions but also by the increasing rate and intensity of these losses which create a cumulative effect that overtaxes the individual's ability to adapt and reintegrate. Management of this problem lies in attempting to control the number of factors that must be dealt with at the same time, finding substitutes for what has been lost and in reminiscing to assist in healthy integration of the past.

Loss is described as the relinquishing of valued internal or external supports that assist the individual in meeting his basic needs. This can become a crisis when it threatens the older person's self-esteem, disrupts his usual lifestyle and cannot be handled in the usual manner of coping (Murray et al, 1980).

Grief

Grief is a subjective emotional and physical response to loss and is the predominant emotion used in mourning. In the grief process, individuals progress through identifiable stages. Kubler-Ross (1969) has described these stages in relation to death as: denial, anger, bargaining, depression and acceptance. These stages are not necessarily linear and some people do not advance through all of them but continually return to one of the early stages. The grief response to losses other than death is a similar process and, depending on the depth of the loss as perceived by the elderly person, it may last for several years.

Factors that impact on grieving include the person's previous experience in dealing with grief and its resultant coping mechanisms (or lack of these), available support systems (persons who are able and willing to assist the person in dealing with grief), and the depth of the loss to the individual.

Depression

Depression is a common occurrence that affects 10-30 percent of the elderly and is often closely associated with physical diseases. Murray (1980) defines depression as an emotional reaction and altered mood state accompanied by a negative self concept and a lowering of self-esteem. It is related in the elderly to the rapid and constant losses that occur and viewed as pathological only when the reactions are excessive in duration and degree.

Burnside (1981) identifies three common types of depression in the elderly: 1) masked depression which is hidden and the person withdraws; 2) reactive depression when the precipitating event or cause is obvious; and 3) depressive states associated with chronic brain syndrome, incipient cerebral arteriosclerosis and Parkinson's disease when the person senses the coming deterioration and fears the future.

A further type of depression is endogenous and is associated with deficiencies in neurotransmitters that conduct impulses across synapses. This type of depression responds to antidepressant drugs.

Blazer (1982) describes the characteristic signs and symptoms of depression as sadness, low mood, pessimism, self criticism, slowed thinking, inability to concentrate, and disturbances in appetite and sleep. This author raises an interesting question on the distinction between depression and demoralization in the elderly person. Demoralization is identified as present when a person is unable to meet demands placed on him by his environment and is unable to escape from this predicament.

TABLE 4-11
Common signs of depression and dementia

Depression	Dementia
Apathy	Onset is slow
Lack of interest in appearance	Dress may indicate general care in
Crying	appearance but inappropriate
No interest in answering questions	Willing to answer questions but answers
	do not make sense
	Screaming

It is important for the nurse to distinguish between depression (which is treatable) and dementia which is progressive and not usually reversible.

The support system available to the elderly person is a crucial factor in managing depression and past coping mechanisms must be identified. Suicide as a coping mechanism for depression is a reality for some elderly who cannot find constructive alternatives. The nurse needs to be aware of the increased rate of suicide, especially in elderly men, and use crisis intervention when appropriate.

Confusion

The incidence of confusion in elderly persons increases with age especially in the decades after 70 and is usually present in diseases related to cerebral functioning. Wolanin and Phillips (1981) define confusion as a disorientation to time and place with incongruous conceptual boundaries, paranormal awareness and verbal statements indicative of memory deficiency. These authors suggest that behaviors related to confusion have cognitive and social implications. Cognitive behaviors are manifested as intellectual deficits whereas social behaviors related to confusion are disruptive and interfere with social functioning. Disease processes, especially those that cause hypoxia, may be identified early by a sudden onset of confusion.

An important distinction to both the elderly person and those responsible for his care is a distinction in the causes of all of the above problems in psychosocial functioning. The cause should be identified and appropriate treatment initiated.

DRUG MANAGEMENT

Responsible drug usage is complex at any age. Persons who have suffered cognitive losses are especially at risk for mismanagement.

For some elderly persons, a variety of factors increase this complexity. These include physiological changes of aging that affect reactions to drugs and an increase in the number of drugs prescribed or used without prescriptions. To assist the elderly person in increasing the effectiveness of drugs taken and decreasing the possibility of detrimental outcomes, the nurse needs to understand geriatric pharmacology and its impact on the individual.

The physiological changes that accompany aging affect the absorption, distribution, metabolism and excretion of drugs that are taken orally (Ivey, 1979). Absorption varies with the status of the individual digestive system. Distribution of drug effects within the body are affected by normal changes in the storage areas for fat and protein. Fat soluble drugs will act less intensely but for a longer period of time than in younger persons since they tend to remain stored in the increased proportion of fat that exists in aging. Lowered serum albumin levels in older persons may affect the distribution of drugs that bind to protein. Changes in the liver function with age affect the metabolism of drugs and may result in unpredictable drug action in an individual. Kidney changes in aging affect the older person's ability to excrete drugs and thus increase the risk of drug toxicity.

The increased incidence of chronic disease in old age increases the probability that one or more drugs will be prescribed for the elderly person. In addition to prescribed drugs, many older people take over-the-counter drugs without sharing this information with the physician who is prescribing for them. Lack of understanding about what a drug should do and what are unwanted side effects can result in inappropriate drug use such as sudden discontinuance without consultation or continued use after the drug has accomplished the desired results.

Some of the common drugs used by the elderly are: drugs for treatment of cardiovascular disease such as digitalis and those used to control arrhythmia, angina, hypertension and blood coagulation; oral insulin for treatment of diabetes; anti-inflammatory drugs commonly used in the treatment of arthritis; analgesics for pain relief; sedatives and hypnotics for control of mental and emotional disturbances; drugs for control of parkinsonian symptoms; antibiotics for infection control and laxatives for bowel problems. Interactions between different drugs or between drugs and food or alcohol consumed often go unnoticed until symptoms are severe. Confusion is a common symptom of drug toxicity but it is often overlooked in the elderly especially if it has been previously noticed due to other causes.

The functional disabilities that occur with increasing frequency in old age can complicate the elderly person's ability to manage the use of drugs. Sensory losses, especially diminished sight, can increase the risk of taking the wrong medication while memory losses can contribute to forgetfulness in taking the needed medicine.

Nursing interventions to assist elderly persons in responsible drug management will include the collaboration of both the individual and the primary caretaker(s). A well-known aid in this undertaking is a written record of each medication being used, the date its use was initiated, its purpose, any side effects to be monitored, potential incompatibility with other drugs or food, and any reactions that have occurred with the individual in the past. Many nurses tape a sample pill on a card with an easily readable label for the drug so that the person taking the drug can easily recognize the pill. The dosage and hours of desired administration are helpful cues when written on the same card.

SUMMARY

Health deviations in the elderly are often treated as primarily physical or primarily psychosocial but the impact of either is relevant to the whole individual and to the society in which he resides. Although deviations are seen as a different entity than normal aging processes, it is recognized that these deviations increase in both number and intensity in the elderly population and must be planned for by both the individual and those responsible for assisting with his care.

References

Abbey, J.C. Aspects of the aging GI tract. In I. Burnside (Ed.), op cit, 1981, 311.

Alcohol and the Elderly. A special report. U.S. Department of Health and Human Services, Public Health Service, Alcohol, Drug Abuse and Mental Health Administration IFS No. 103, December 31, 1982.

Atwood, J. Cardiovascular problems. In D. Carnevali and M. Patrick (Eds.), *Nursing management for the elderly.* Philadelphia: J.B. Lippincott Co., 1979, 247.

Bartol, M. and Heitkemper, M. Gastrointestinal problems. In D. Carnevali and M. Patrick (Eds.), op cit, 311, 324.

Bither, S., Respiratory problems. In D. Carnevali and M. Patrick (Eds.), op cit, 427.

Blainey, C. Diabetes Mellitus. In D. Carnevali and M. Patrick (Eds.), op cit, 308.

Blazer, D.G. *Depression in late life.* St. Louis: The C.V. Mosby Co., 1982.

Bruno, P. Skin problems. In D. Carnevali and M. Patrick (Eds.), op cit, 469.

Burnside, I.M. *Nursing and the aged.* New York: McGraw-Hill Book Co., 1981.

Butler, R.N. and Lewis, M. *Aging and mental health* (3rd ed.). St. Louis: The C.V. Mosby Co., 1982.

Carnevali, D.L. and Patrick M. *Nursing management for the elderly.* Philadelphia: J.B. Lippincott Co., 1979.

Carty, R. Patients who cannot hear. *Nursing Forum,* 1972, *11*(3), 290-299.

Eliopoulos, C. *Gerontological nursing.* New York: Harper & Row, 1979.

Field, M.A. Urinary incontinence in the elderly: An overview. *Journal of Gerontological Nursing.* New York: Harper & Row, 1979.

Goldman, R. Aging changes in structure and function. In D. Carnevali and M. Patrick (Eds.), op cit, 73.

Ivey, M. Drug use. In D. Carnevali and M. Patrick (Eds.), op cit, 169.

Kubler-Ross, E. *On death and dying.* New York: MacMillan Publishing Co., 1969.

Molbo, D.M., Cancer. In D. Carnevali and M. Patrick (Eds.), op cit, 207-245.

Murray, R., Heulskoetler, M., and O'Driscoll, D. *The nursing process in later maturity.* Englewood Cliffs, NJ: Prentice-Hall, Inc., 1980.

Preston, C. Losses of Aging. In D. Carnevali and M. Patrick (Eds.), op cit, 515-521.

Progress Report on Senile Dementia of the Alzheimer's Type. National Institute on Aging. NIH Publication No. 81, 6-2343, September 1981.

Roberts, S. Cardiopulmonary abnormalities in aging. In I. Burnside (Ed.), op cit, 1981, 236.

Rockstein, M. and Sussman, M. *Biology of aging.* Belmont, CA: Wadsworth Publishing Co., 1979.

Shanck, A. Musculoskeletal problems in aging. In I. Burnside (Ed.), op cit, 1981, 284.

Thomas, E.G. Application of stress factors in gerontologic nursing. *Nursing Clinics of North America, 14*(4), December 1979, 607-620.

Wolanin, M.O. and Phillips, L.R.F. *Confusion: Prevention and care.* St. Louis: The C.V. Mosby Co., 1981.

Suggested Readings on Deviations in Health Common to the Aging Process

Alford, D.M. and Moll, J.A. Helping elderly patients in ambulatory settings cope with drug therapy. *Nursing Clinics of North America,* 1982, *17,* 275-282.

Aloia, G.F. Exercise and skeletal health. *Journal of the American Geriatrics Society,* 1981, XXIX(3), 104-107.

Barney, J.L. and Neukom, J.E. Use of Arthritis care by the elderly. *The Gerontologist,* 1979, *19*(6), 548-554.

Dohrenwend, B. and Dohrenwend, B. (Eds.), *Stressful life events: Their nature and effects.* New York: Wiley & Co., 1974.

Gaeta, M. and Gaetano, R. *The elderly: Their health and the drugs in their lives.* Dubuque, IA: Kendall/Hunt Publishing Co., 1977.

Glenner, G. Alzheimer's disease (senile dementia): A research update and critique with recommendations. *Journal of the American Geriatrics Society, 30*(1), 1982, 59-62.

Goldman, R. Aging of the excretory system: Kidney and bladder. In C. Finsh and L. Hayflick (Eds.), *Handbook of the Biology of Aging.* Van Nostrand Reinhold, New York, 1977.

Goldman, R. Aging changes in structure and function. In D. Carnevali and M. Patrick (Eds.), *Nursing management for the elderly.* Philadelphia: J.B. Lippincott Co., 1979.

Hartford, J. and Samorajski, T. Alcoholism in the geriatric population. *Journal of the American Geriatrics Society, 30*(1), 1982, 18-24.

Kim, K. and Grier, M. Pacing effects of medication instruction for the elderly. *Journal of Gerontological Nursing,* 7, 1981, 464-468.

Lamy, P. *Prescribing for the elderly.* Littleton: PSG Publishing Co., Inc., 1980.

Lawton, M.P. Psychosocial and environmental approaches to the care of senile dementia patients. In J. Cole and J.E. Barrett (Eds.), *Psychopathology in the Aged.* New York: Raven Press, 1982, 265-280.

Mackey, A. OBS and nursing care. *Journal of Gerontological Nursing, 9*(2), 1983, 74-85.

Moss, F.E. and Halamandaris. *Too old too sick too bad.* Germantown, MD: Aspen Systems Corp., 1977.

Ouslander, J.G. et. al. Urinary incontinence in elderly nursing home patients. *Journal of the American Medical Association.* September 10, 1982, Vol. 248, No. 10, 1194-1198.

Pagliaro, L. and Pagliaro, A. *Pharmacologic Aspects of Aging.* St. Louis: C.V. Mosby Co., 1983.

Parkes, C.M. *Bereavement: Studies of grief in adult life.* New York: International Universities Press, 1972.

Peterson, J.A. Social-psychological aspects of death and dying. In J.E. Birren and R.B. Sloane (Eds.), *Handbook of mental health and aging.* Englewood Cliffs, NJ: Prentice-Hall, Inc., 1980, 922-942.

Potempa, K. and Roberts, K.V. Cardiovascular drugs and the older adult. *Nursing Clinics of North America*, 1982, *17*, 263-274.

Skillman, T.G. Can osteoporosis be prevented? *Geriatrics*, February 1980, 95-102.

Susser, M. Ethical components in the definition of health. *International Journal of Health Services*, *4*, 1974, 535-548.

Vestal, R.F. Pharmacology and aging. *Journal of the American Geriatrics Association*, 1982, *30*, 191-200.

Vogel, C. Anxiety and depression among the elderly. *Journal of Gerontological Nursing*, *8*(4), 1982, 213-216.

5

Support Systems for the Elderly

As more people are living longer and managing the impairments of age as well as the problems of chronic illness, they increasingly need support systems to assist them in maintaining health and well-being. The concept of extended support systems is a universal one reflecting the various cultures in many societies. Older adults have usually contributed to the support of many others during their lifetime and when illness and/or aging diminish their capacity to meet their needs independently they are dependent on others for varying degrees of assistance in managing their lives and their environment. In a report presented to the U.S. House of Representatives Select Committee on Aging (Every Ninth American, 1982), twenty percent of the non-institutionalized elderly (age sixty-five and over) were described as needing some form of regular assistance in maintaining health and functions of daily living.

Support systems for the elderly are similar to those available to all ages. They include families, friends and community resources. Families continue to provide the major support system for most elderly. The guardians of social policy that involves support systems in the U.S. today are concerned with the shift in family patterns and the concurrent rise in life expectancy. If this combination in the demographic trend continues, it will result in more elderly persons needing more support from families that are smaller in numbers and contain fewer members that are able and available for the care of elderly persons. Increased assistance to existing family resources and provision of additional community and professional resources seem inevitable. This chapter will discuss both family and community support systems for the elderly and nursing implications based on these supports.

FAMILIES AS SUPPORT SYSTEMS

Less than five percent of older Americans do not have families (Shanas, first 1979 entry). The structure and the functioning pattern of these families differ but the responsibility of families to care for and socialize children and to provide security for adults is generally accepted. A 1975 survey of non-institutional community aged showed immediate family — husbands, wives, children — to be the major social support during illness and this support was the factor that allowed persons to stay out of institutions. A primary need of the elderly was for regular and concerned visitors. The quality of the visits was seen as more important than the number of visitors and this quality role was generally assumed by relatives. This pattern reflected a mutual expectation between generations and in families.

Spouse support to elderly persons is influenced by sex-related differences in aging married persons. In 1978, for every 100 older men there were 146 older women. Seventy-eight percent of the older men were married with one-third of these having wives under 65 years of age. Fifty-two percent of older women were widows and there were five widows for every widower (Facts about older Americans). The increase in divorce rates for all age groups will further affect these demographic facts. It seems unlikely that there will be a major shift in the proportion of men and women in this age group and thus there will continue to be more women needing care.

In a recent study by Vinick (1982), husbands who had cared for disabled wives before their deaths were interviewed and results suggest that these men had been able to adapt to the caretaking role and were able to provide needed support. It is interesting to note that in this sample of twenty-five there was a significant negative correlation between having cared for a sick wife and the desire to remarry with caretaking husbands less willing to consider marriage.

Wives who provide the primary care for elderly husbands were described in studies by Fengler and Goodrich (1979) as the hidden patients. A model for supportive services for older women caring for disabled spouses was developed by Crossman, London and Barry (1981).

Daughters have been identified as a main support of elderly mothers (Treas, 1977). A decrease in the number of unmarried women in the population of available daughters and an increase in the number of daughters who hold jobs outside their homes are two factors that have impacted on the availability of daughters to provide for elderly mothers especially if substantial personal care is needed. Treas has also described the influence of economic changes on the relationship between the generations. Increased income for both generations has liberated them from total economic dependency on each other but the care of an elderly family member remains an economic burden for families. Further descriptions of the roles which daughters fulfill in the care of elderly widowed mothers are provided by Shanas (1980) and Brody (1981).

The concept of filial responsibility expectations was investigated by Seelbach and Sauer (1977) and measured against parental morale in elderly parents. They found levels of filial responsibility expectations significantly and inversely associated with parental morale levels. These findings raise questions on the differences in how filial responsibility is perceived from one generation to the next.

Sussman (1965) described affective and social support as more important to aging parents than economic assistance. This concept lends importance to the idea that economic support from the community may be needed to free adult children from this burden and allow them to concentrate on providing needed

...pport. Families often maintain contact with elderly relatives after
... to nursing homes even though these visits are not pleasant and the
...ay seek needed emotional support from staff members. Nurses can
...amilies at this difficult time by listening to their concerns, helping them
... rt the myths of aging from the realities, giving appropriate referrals for
needed community services and supporting the self-esteem of the family
members.

The myth that elderly people are being abandoned by their families is
exploded in the facts presented by Shanas (second 1979 entry). Eighty percent
of the elderly have living children. In 1975, eighteen percent of these elderly
lived in the same household with one of these children, while another thirty-four
percent of these elderly lived within ten minutes distance of a child. Siblings are
another source of support for the elderly and eighty percent of the elderly have
living brothers and sisters. Elderly persons turn first to family, then to neighbors
or friends, and only as a last resort do they turn to formal sources of assistance
such as community resources, churches and health agencies. Families that do
not feel able to meet demands of elderly members will turn to community agencies for support.

COMMUNITY SUPPORT SYSTEMS FOR THE ELDERLY

Community supports for the elderly vary widely. Geriatric Day Care centers are being developed in many parts of the country to provide care for elderly
persons who need assistance during the day when other family members are
unavailable.

Senior citizen centers, some with nutrition programs, are also available in
various locations. Recreation centers and various park services offer programs
for the well elderly. Education departments as well as community colleges and
universities have special programs available for the elderly. The American
Association of Retired Persons and similar private organizations offer a variety
of programs specific to the elderly.

Home care services are available for those who require this type of service.
Visiting nurses and other health professionals can provide care including physical therapy, nutrition counselling and social services. Aides and homemakers
are available for supplementary service.

Respite care offers temporary institutional care for relief to families who
need rest from the continual care of the impaired elderly. Senior citizen residences
provide a supportive environment that may include one or more meals daily in a
central dining room, environmental adjustments such as rails and ramps to
assist in mobility, and ready access to needed assistance on a twenty-four hour
basis. In life care communities, these types of support services are supplemented
by intermediate and skilled care units and elderly persons who reside there can
utilize these services as needed without necessarily giving up their individual apartments.

The existence of the above mentioned community support systems, and any more that are not mentioned, is not equated with their availability to populations who need them. They represent an ideal rather than a real description of services for most communities, and when they are available, they are not always accessible due to problems of transportation, acceptability to the elderly person and cost.

The development of various support systems for elderly persons is a societal step in the right direction. Follow-up of needed supports to link the elderly person with the appropriate services, and available funding for individuals and families who cannot afford to pay are essential if society is to continue in a positive direction.

NURSING IMPLICATIONS IN SUPPORT SYSTEMS

The nurse who is involved in gerontology has both an active and a referent role in support systems. The referent role is that of 1) keeping current with support systems available in the community, 2) evaluating their quality and, 3) being knowledgeable on how to utilize these systems. The active role is in collaborating with the existing support systems to assist the elderly in promoting, maintaining and regaining their health, and when appropriate, assisting with the dying process.

Providing nursing services to families as well as to individuals has historically been an essential component in public health nursing practice. The current emphasis on primary care nursing has extended the emphasis on family centered nursing into acute care settings. Professionals in health care and aging often meet a disproportionate number of elderly who lack family as a support system and this has sometimes resulted in both professional and policy emphasis that does not incorporate the family as an essential resource for the elderly. The remaining section of this chapter will describe some of the existing efforts in gerontological nursing to assure the inclusion of the family or other caretaker in the process of nursing care.

Consideration of the family role in the nursing care of the elderly is described by Reinhardt and Quinn (1979), Murray et al (1980), Ebersole (1981) and Burnside (1981). Each of these nursing texts stresses the importance of the family in working with the elderly and Burnside emphasizes the importance of assessing the home including physical environment, interpersonal relationships, physical and psychological dynamics, and defense mechanisms as a basis for assessing what services are needed (p. 437).

Freeman and Heinrich (1981) highlight family health nursing care for the aging family and present a tool to be used as a basis for estimating the nursing needs of a family. This tool is called the Family Coping Index and encourages nurses to view the family coping ability in specific areas not only in its present state but with the added dimension of a future expected state, for better or for

worse. In this tool, a nursing need is seen as present when:
1. there is a health problem with which the family cannot cope, and
2. it is likely that nursing will make a difference in the family's coping ability.

The following areas of function are assessed with emphasis on nursing intervention:

Physical independence
Therapeutic competence
Knowledge of health condition
Application of principles of general hygiene
Health attitudes
Emotional competence
Family living
Physical environment
Use of community facilities

Although this tool was not designed specifically for the family with an elderly member, it is a helpful assessment tool for use in these families. A family assessment tool specific to elderly persons was not found in the literature.

Appropriate nursing intervention to the elderly and their families in the home can enable families to keep their elderly members within the family system without neglecting the needs of the family as a unit. Accomplishing this balance between all family members is challenging and, depending on the extent of need and the existence of resources, financial as well as professional support may be needed.

The 1981 White House Conference on Aging recommended both alternative forms of care for the elderly and a new program of research on the care of caregivers such as the family members. The first World Assembly on Aging, sponsored by the United Nations in Vienna in July, 1982, presented an international round table on "The Family as a Source of Support for the Elderly". This round table was chaired by Virginia Little, a well-known nursing expert from the United States. Recommendations from the group included the need for more research on the internal socio-psychological structure of the family and intergenerational exchanges. The challenge to provide care for the elderly has been identified nationally and internationally. The use of many support systems will assist in this goal. The challenge to the gerontological nurse is to be aware of these systems and to continue to advance the participation of nursing within these systems.

SUMMARY

The efforts of elderly persons to maintain their health and well-being often require support from others. Families provide a large amount of this support. Community services for the elderly can assist them and their families. Nurses working with elderly persons need to be aware of how to collaborate with both the individuals and their families to utilize appropriate community services.

References

Brody, E.M. Women in the middle and family help to older people. *The Gerontologist*, 1981, *21*(5), 471-480.

Burnside, I.M. *Nursing and the aged*. New York: McGraw-Hill Book Co., 1981, 437.

Crossman, L., London, C., and Barry, C. Older women caring for disabled spouses: A model for supportive services. *The Gerontologists*, 1981, *21*, 464-470.

Ebersole, P. and Hess, P. *Toward healthy aging*. St. Louis: C.V. Mosby and Co., 1981.

Fengler, A.P. and Goodrich, W. Wives of elderly disabled men: The hidden patients. *The Gerontologist*, 1979, *19*, 175-183.

Freeman, R. and Heinrich, J. *Community health nursing practice*. Philadelphia: W.B. Saunders Co., 1981, 226, 555.

House of Representatives Select Committee on Aging. *Every ninth American* (1982 ed.), Washington, DC: U.S. Government Printing Office, 1982.

Murray, R., Huelskoetter, M. and O'Driscoll, D. *The nursing process in later maturity*. Englewood Cliffs, NJ: Prentice-Hall, Inc., 1980.

Reinhardt, A. and Quinn, M. *Current practice in gerontological nursing*. St. Louis: C.V. Mosby Co., 1979.

Seelback, W.C. and Sauer, Wm.J. Filial responsibility expectations and morale among aged parents. *The Gerontologist*, (December), *17*(6), 492-499.

Shanas, E. The family as a social support system in old age. *The Gerontologist*, 1979, *19*(2).

Shanas, E. Social myth as hypotheses: The case of the family relations of old people. *The Gerontologist*, 1979, *19*(3).

Shanas, E. Older people and their families: The new pioneers. *Journal of Marriage and the Family*, 1980, *42*, 9-15.

Treas, J. Family support systems for the aged. *The Gerontologist*, December 1977, *17*(6), 486-491.

U.S. Department of Health and Human Services, Office of Human Development Services Administration on Aging, Pub. No. 80-20006. *Facts about older Americans*, 1979.

Vinick, B. Elderly men as caretakers of wives. Paper given in Boston, Annual Meeting of the Gerontological Society of America, November 1982.

Suggested Readings on Support Systems for the Elderly

Aronson, M. and Lipkowitz, R. Senile dementia, Alzheimer's type: The family and the health care delivery system. *Journal of the American Geriatrics Society*, 1981, *29*(12), 568-571.

Barnes, R., Raskind, M., Scott, M., and Murphy, C. Problems of families caring for Alzheimer patients: Use of a support group. *Journal of the American Geriatrics Society*, 1981 *29*(2), 80-85.

Bengtson, V.L., Olander, E.B., and Haddad, A.A. The "generation gap" and aging family members: Toward a conceptual model. In J.E. Gubrium (Ed.), *Time, roles and self in old age*. Human Sciences Press, New York, 1976.

Blazer, D.G. and Siegler, I. *Working with the family of the older adult*. Menlo Park, CA: Addison Wesley, 1981.

Branch, L. and Jette, E. Elders use of informal long term care assistance. *The Gerontologist*, February 1983, *23*(1), 51-56.

Brody, E.G. The aging family. *Gerontologist*, 1966, *6*, 201-206.

Brody, E.M. *Long term care of older people*. A practical guide, 1977.

Brody, S., Poulshock, S.W. and Masciocchi, C. The family caring unit: A major consideration in the long term support system. *Gerontologist*, 1978, *18*, 556-561.

Clements, I.W. and Buchanan, D.M. (Eds.). *Family therapy - a nursing perspective*. New York: John Wiley and Sons, 1982.

Eyde, D.R. and Rich, J.A. *Psychological distress in aging: A family management model.* Rockville, MD: Aspen Publications, 1983.

Gwyther, L. and Matteson, M. Care for the caregivers. *Journal of Gerontological Nursing,* 1983, *9*(2), 92-95.

Herr, J.J. and Weakland, J.H. *Counseling elders and their families.* New York: Springer Publishing Co., 1979.

Mace, N. and Rabins, P. *The 36-Hour Day.* Baltimore: The Johns Hopkins University Press, 1981.

MacVicar, M.G. and Archbold, P. A framwork for family assessment in chronic illness. *Nursing Forum,* 1976, *15*(2), 180-194.

Mindel, C.J. and Wright, R. Satisfaction in multigenerational households. *Journal of Gerontology,* 1982, *37*(4), 483-489.

Orbach, H.L. Symposium: Aging, families, and family relations. Behavioral and social science perspectives on our knowledge, our myths, and our research. *The Gerontologist,* February 1983, *23*(1), 24-25.

Rauseo, L. Separation of generations - who benefits? *Journal of Gerontological Nursing,* January/February 1977, *3*(1), 40-41.

Shanas, E. and Sussman, M.B. (Eds.). *Family, bureaucracy and the elderly.* Durham, NC: Duke University Press, 1977.

Strieb, G. The frail elderly: Research dilemmas and research opportunities. *The Gerontologist,* February 1983, *23*(1), 40-44.

Sussman, M.B. Relationship of adult children with their parents in the United States. In E. Shanas and G. Streib (Eds.), *Social structure and the family: Generational relations.* Englewood Cliffs, NJ: Prentice-Hall, 1965.

Sussman, M.B. The family life of old people. In R.H. Binstock and E. Shanas (Eds.), *Handbook of aging and the social sciences.* New York: Van Nostrand Reinhold, 1977, 218-243.

Troll, L.E., Miller, S.J., and Atchley, R.C. *Families in later life.* Belmont, CA: Wadsworth, 1979.

6

Process in Gerontological Nursing

T he nursing process, a functional concept utilized in practice and taught in curriculum, is similar to the problem-solving process used in other scientific endeavors and in research.

The general thrust of the nursing process is that we need to know where we are, where we are going, how to get there, and how to recognize when we have arrived. For purposes of this chapter, the "we" refers to the elderly client (and caretakers when appropriate) and the nurse who is providing the primary nursing care and/or has assumed the responsibility for the nursing process. The terms for the steps in this process are commonly identified in the nursing literature as assessing, planning, implementing and evaluating (Yura and Walsh, 1978).

ASSESSING: OR 'WHERE ARE WE?'

A comprehensive assessment of where the elderly person is in relation to health can be based on many of the factors described in this monograph and elsewhere. Theoretical foundations include assessment of developmental and psychosocial factors that are influencing the person's aging. Biophysical attributes that influence health and illness need careful assessment. Support systems will define the social situation in which the elderly person operates and a functional assessment will determine how the person is able to integrate existing resources into activities of daily living. Both the positive and negative dimensions of the above mentioned aspects of the person's life are important. The existing level of health and function is essential to give true meaning to the level of health deviation and dysfunction. Existing strengths and helpful past coping mechanisms are balanced out with problems and deficits in function for assessment purposes.

To assist in assessing elderly persons who may need nursing care, a number of tools have been developed. Schrock (1980) describes an assessment tool that includes physical, cultural, psychological, social, and economic factors. Data are subjective since they focus on the client's view of his condition as told to the nurse. The categories of data included in the tool are: demographic, health-illness, psychological health, economic resource, and cultural and social. In addition to gathering this information, the nurse is expected to utilize skills in physical examination and observation to complete the assessment.

Mezey et al (1980) describe the health assessment of the older person in relationship to an interview which consists of obtaining a general health history, an assessment of various systems that includes both history and physical examination, and the development of a client profile. These authors additionally describe community and home assessments that can be related to both the needs and resources of the elderly person. The community assessment describes overall features, population characteristics, service facilities and environmental/safety conditions. The home assessment guide describes roles and relationships, comfort and convenience, and safety factors. This approach, which combines the characteristics of the individual with those of the environment in which he dwells, represents a broad view of health assessment.

Lantz (1980) has described an assessment tool that is designed to provide a basis for beginning individualized care. It includes vital statistics, physical parameters, psychological parameters, and sociological parameters. Physical assessment of the gerontological client is described by Carotenuto and Bullock (1980) with a focus on problem-oriented format. Understanding this orientation of assessment is crucial for communication with our colleagues in the medical profession and for operationalizing interdisciplinary efforts in the care of the elderly in acute care settings where problem-oriented records are used.

Wolanin (1981) has described a nursing assessment model for use with elderly persons that is based on the FANCAP tool developed by Abbey. This has been modified to FANCAPES and includes assessment of fluids, aeration, nutrition, communication, activity, pain, elimination, and social skills. Wolanin adds one further dimension in assessing the elderly — the clients' perception of their own health status and their attitude toward dying and death. Panicucci (1983) has discussed the use of the functional assessment model in nursing care of the elderly in the acute care setting. She has identified three general levels of function: a) control over body, b) control over home environment, and c) ability to function independently in an interdependent world.

All of these assessment tools and many others that are being used by nurses today are valuable as guides for organizing needed information in making an assessment of an elderly client. They need to be modified, adapted, expanded or contracted based on the specific situation in which care is being delivered. The nurse is not always the primary caregiver or even the person with responsibility for planning the care. The repertoire of professional nurses has expanded into highly sophisticated areas of health care delivery. Accompanying this expansion must be a good measure of common sense as to when interventions are appropriate to use. The nurse who finds herself one of a small number of nurses on the staff of a nursing home where the primary job responsibilities are defined in areas of medication dispensing or managerial functioning needs to establish priorities that will promote good patient care. In such a situation, nursing intervention may be focused on impacting on the available care through working with others in the system and providing a role model for gerontologic nursing. Shine and Kopac (1982) have described a curriculum guide that assists nurses in this function.

PLANNING: OR 'WHERE ARE WE GOING?'

Let us assume that we have access to a thorough assessment and that the work situation allows us to exercise our talent in using the nursing process with a gerontological client. The question of where we are going becomes crucial. This is the planning stage of the process and includes both general goals and specific objectives. The goals will guide the direction and can be broad and encompassing. The objectives, by contrast, need to be well defined and specific. They will serve as activators for a working plan and also as criteria for subsequent evaluation.

Mr. J may want to "return to his normal activities" — a goal. Assessment will have determined what these activities are and what existing factors are available in Mr. J and in the system around him to enable him to reach this goal. It is at this point in the nursing process that the nurse may have to deal with some of the unpleasant realities that occur with increasing frequency in the aged when they can no longer resume the same activities as they had been involved in previously. If Mr. J. previously gardened extensively in his yard and has recently lost his leg due to peripheral vascular complications, some modification of normal activities will be required at least for a period of time. With assistance for his personal needs from health care providers, such as medical, physiotherapy, nursing and nutritional staff, and assistance from others in his support system who can compensate for his lack of mobility such as family members, friends, and neighbors, he would be able to enjoy sitting in his yard or planting in a raised plot or a window box. The challenge would be to focus on realistic goals that would offer some opportunity for hope and joy while allowing Mr. J the expression of appropriate grief for those functions which he has lost. After dealing with this needed adjustment, the nurse and Mr. J could develop both goals and objectives that are mutually acceptable and attainable.

Objectives that would define where we are going might be identified under the adapted goal as follows: a) within two months, Mr. J will spend one hour each day in the garden working with plants; b) in three months, Mr. J will walk with a prosthesis . . . etc. It is important that the objectives be defined in terms of what Mr. J will be able to do, under what conditions, and in what time period. This type of specificity, when possible, keeps both the client and the caretakers functionally oriented and keeps the focus on normalcy rather than on the illness. Evaluation is easier when behaviors to be achieved are well defined.

IMPLEMENTING: 'HOW DO WE GET THERE?'

This phase follows the decision making on goals and objectives described above. It involves further decision making and objectives, but these are the objectives relative to the process rather than the outcome and they describe the activities that are deemed necessary to accomplish the goals and objectives. The motivation of the client was perhaps the most crucial component in deciding where to go, with the nurse offering support. In this phase, the crucial element may well be that of the professional "know-how" and judgment of the nurse in knowing about needed activities and resources, knowing how to access these support systems and enabling Mr. J to utilize them.

To implement the mutually agreed upon plan, it will be necessary for the health team, including the patient, to do a variety of activities associated with convalescence. These include arranging for appointments with the physiotherapist, doing regular range of motion exercises, eating nourishing meals regularly, as well as some activities that are specific to what Mr. J wants to accomplish such as reviewing the current seed catalogues, talking with the local storekeeper and arranging a location that he can reach for his planting activities. The scope and variety of these activities will require help from family and friends — all of this is not within the realm of the nurse, but communication with the others who will assist Mr. J is essential to assure the implementation of the nursing process.

EVALUATING: OR 'HOW DO WE KNOW WE HAVE ARRIVED?'

The evaluation stage of the nursing process is crucial, not only to the client who values the results and the nurse who receives personal and professional satisfaction from it, but also to the third party payers who fund nursing care. Whether it is the hospital or agency that employs the nurse as a staff member, the insurance company who reimburses the nurse and/or her employer for services rendered, the client who pays the nurse directly, or the home care or private duty agency, there is need to justify that quality of the product we call nursing care.

There are usually at least two layers of evaluation to be considered — the ultimate outcome, and the process that was used. These are under our categories of where we were going and how we were getting there. Evaluation focused on patient outcomes is concerned with whether we got where we were going, thus accentuating the importance of clearly defining the goals. Evaluation focused on the process looks at whether we did the activities we identified as essential to how we were going to get there. Both types of evaluation are appropriate and, if well done, can provide important evidence on the value of professional nursing care.

SUMMARY

The nursing process is an important tool in the delivery of professional nursing care. The organization of needed data may vary with the format chosen. This choice is guided by the specific circumstances in which the nursing process is being used. Whatever the format, the process includes answers to the questions of where we are, where we are going, how we will get there, and how we will evaluate both the outcome and the process.

References

Carotenute, R. and Bullock, J. *Physical assessment of the gerontologic client.* Philadelphia: F.A. Davis Co., 1980.

Freeman, R. and Heinrich, J. *Community health nursing practice.* Philadelphia: W.B. Saunders Co., 1981.

Lantz, J. Assessment: A beginning to individualized care. In Edna M. Stillwell (Ed.), *Readings in gerontological nursing.* New Jersey: Charles B. Slack, Inc., 1980.

Mezey, M.D., Rauckhorst, L.H., and Stokes, S.A. *Health assessment of the older individual.* New York: Springer Publishing Co., 1980.

Orem, D. *Nursing: Concepts of practice* (2nd ed.). New York: McGraw-Hill Book Co., 1980.

Panicucci, C. Functional assessment of the Older Adult in the Acute Care Setting. *Nursing Clinics of North America.* Vol. 18, No. 2, June 1983, 355-363.

Schrock, M. *Holistic assessment of the healthy aged.* New York: John Wiley and Sons, 1980.

Wolanin, M.O. The nursing assessment. In Irene Burnside (Ed.), *Nursing and the aged* (2nd ed.). New York: McGraw-Hill Book Co., 1981.

Yura, H. and Walsh, M.B. *The nursing process: Assessing, planning, implementing, and evaluating* (3rd ed.). New York: Appleton-Century-Crofts, 1978.

Suggested Readings on Nursing Process in Gerontological Nursing

Burnside, I.M., Ebersole, P., and Monea, H.E. (Eds.). *Psychosocial caring throughout the life span.* New York: McGraw-Hill Book Co., 1979.

Burnside, I.M. *Nursing and the aged.* New York: McGraw-Hill Book Co., 1981.

Carnevali, D.L. and Patrick, M. *Nursing management for the elderly.* Philadelphia: J.B. Lippincott Co., 1979.

Ebersole, P. and Hess, P. *Toward healthy aging.* St. Louis: C.V. Mosby Co., 1981.

Eliopoulos, C. Assessment and action in gerontological nursing. *Family and community health,* April 1978, *1,* 80-81.

Eliopoulos, C. *Gerontological nursing.* New York: Harper & Row, 1979.

Feeley, E., Shine, M., and Sloboda, S. *Fundamentals of nursing care.* New York: D. Van Nostrand Co., 1980.

Futrell, M., Brovender, S., McKinnon-Mullett, E., and Brower, J.T. *Primary health care of the older adult.* North Scituate, MA: Duxbury Press, 1980.

Golander, H. and Bergman, R. Evaluation of care for the aged: A multipurpose guide. *Journal of Advanced Nursing,* 1982, *1,* 203-210.

Lantz, J. Assessment: A beginning to individualized care. In Edna M. Stillwell (Ed.), *Readings in gerontological nursing.* New York: Charles B. Slack, Inc., 1980.

Murray, R., Huelskoetler, M., and O'Driscoll, D. *The nursing process in later maturity.* Englewood Cliffs, NJ: Prentice-Hall, Inc., 1980.

Phillips, B.R., Baster, R.G., and Stephens, S.A. Approach to the client assessment instrument for the national long term care demonstration evaluation. (Draft) Princeton, NJ: Mathematica Policy Research, January 1981.

Quinn, J.L. and Ryan, N.E. Assessment of the older adult: A "Holistic" approach. *Journal of Gerontological Nursing,* March/April 1979, *1*(2), 13-18.

Reinhardt, A. and Quinn, M. *Current practice in gerontological nursing.* St. Louis: C.V. Mosby Co., 1979.

Rogers, J.C. Advocacy: The key to assessing the older client. *Journal of Gerontological Nursing.* January 1980, *6*(1), 33-36.

Shine, M.S. and Kopac, C. Gerontological Nursing: A Current Curriculum Guide for Registered Nurses in Long Term Care Facilities. Washington, DC: The American Health Care Association, 1982.

Yurick, A.G., Robb, S.S., Spier, B.E., and Ebert, N.J. *The aged person and the nursing process.* New York: Appleton-Century-Crofts, 1980.

A PPENDIX 1

ANA Standards of Gerontological Nursing Practice

STANDARD 1

Data are systematically and continuously collected about the health status of the older adult. The data are accessible, communicated, and recorded.

Rationale: In order to provide comprehensive nursing care of the older adult, the data are collected from a framework that includes the scientific findings and knowledge derived from the fields of gerontology and nursing.

Assessment Factors

1.   Health status data includes the older adult:
     Normal responses to the aging process
     Physiological, psychological, sociological and ecological status
     Modes of communication
     Individual's patterns of coping
     Prior life-style
     Independent performance of activities of everyday living
     Perception of and satisfaction with current health status
     Health goals
     Human material resources available and accessible
2.   Health status data are collected from:
     The older adult, significant others, health care personnel
     Older individuals in the immediate environment who are involved
        in the care of the older adult
     Interviews, examinations, observation, records and reports
3.   The data are:
     Accessible on the older adult's records
     Retrievable from record-keeping system
     Communicated to those responsible for the older adult's care
     Accurate
     Confidential

STANDARD 2

Nursing diagnoses are derived from the identified normal responses of the individual to aging and the data collected about the health status of the older adult.

Rationale: Each person ages in an individual way. The individual's normal responses to aging must be identified before deviations in response requiring nursing actions can be identified.

Assessment Factors

1.   The older adult's health status is compared to the norm, and a determination is made regarding deviations from the norm.
2.   The older adult's prior life-style, responses to the aging process, and personal goals and objectives are identified.
3.   The older adult's strengths and limitations are identified.
4.   The nursing diagnosis is related to and congruent with the diagnosis and plan of all other professionals caring for the older adult.

STANDARD 3

A plan of nursing care is developed in conjunction with the older adult and/ or significant others that includes goals derived from the nursing diagnosis.

Rationale: Goals are a determination of the results to be achieved and are an essential part of planning care. All goals are ultimately directed toward maximizing achievable independence in everyday living.

Assessment Factors

1.   Goals are congruent with other planned therapies, are stated in realistic and measurable terms, and are assigned a time period for achievement.
2.   Goals determine specific nursing approaches that will promote, maintain and restore health.
3.   Goals are measured by the eventual outcomes of nursing care.
4.   The established goals incorporate:
      Normal developmental processes of aging
      Individuality of the older adult
      Needs for intimacy and sexual expression
      Slowing down
      Losses
      Adaptability

STANDARD 4

The plan of nursing care includes the priorities and the prescribed nursing approaches and measures to achieve the goals derived from the nursing diagnosis.

Rationale: Priorities and approaches are an integral part of the planning process and are necessary to the successful achievement of the goals.

Assessment Factors

1. Physical and psychosocial measures are planned to prevent, ameliorate, or control specific problems of the older adult and are related to the nursing diagnosis and goals of care.
2. Environmental hazards, which may include high-frequency sounds, glaring surfaces, and overproduction of stimuli that cause confusion are eliminated.
3. Methods of adaptation using concepts of wellness are taught to the older adult.
4. Specific approaches are identified to orient the older adult to new roles and relationships, to any new surroundings, and to relevant health sources.
5. Specific approaches are identified to promote social interactions and effective communication.

STANDARD 5

The plan of care is implemented, using appropriate nursing actions.
Rationale: Appropriate nursing actions are purposefully directed toward the stated goals.

Assessment Factors

1. Nursing actions are:
    Consistent with plan of care developed in collaboration with the older adult and with appropriate input from other health disciplines
    Based on scientific principles
    Individualized to the specific situation
    Modified to allow for alternative approaches
    Used to provide a safe and therapeutic environment
    Compatible with the physiological, psychological, and social data acquired
    Task-delegated as deemed appropriate
    Planned to meet specific criteria as described in protocols

STANDARD 6

The older adult and/or significant others participate in determining the progress attained in the achievement of established goals.
Rationale: The older adult and/or significant others are essential components in the determination of nursing's impact on the individual's health status.

Assessment Factors

1. Current data are used to measure progress toward goal achievement.
2. Nursing actions are analyzed for effectiveness in goal achievement.
3. The older adult and/or significant others evaluate nursing actions and goal achievement.
4. Plans for the nursing follow-up of the older adult are made to permit the ongoing assessment of the effects of nursing care.

STANDARD 7

The older adult and/or significant others participate in the on-going process of assessment, the setting of new goals, the reordering of priorities, the revision of plans for nursing care, and the initiation of new nursing actions.

Rationale: Comprehensive nursing care is dependent upon actively involving the older adult and/or significant others in a continuing dynamic process.

Assessment Factors

1. Assessment is based on the level of progress of the older adult in goal achievement.
2. The older adult and/or significant others assist in the identification of new goals and the reordering of priorities.
3. Plans are updated and revised.
4. New nursing actions are appropriately initiated.

American Nurses' Association Division on Gerontological Nursing Practice. *Standards of Gerontological Nursing Practice.* Kansas City, MO: The Association, 1976.

*A*PPENDIX 2

ANA Code of Ethics for Nurses

1. Provision of services with respect for human dignity and individual uniqueness regardless of social or economic status, personal attributes, or health problems.
2. Safeguarding of the client's right to privacy and protection of confidential information.
3. Safeguarding the client and the public if health and safety are affected by the incompetent, unethical, or illegal practice of any person.
4. Assuming responsibility and accountability for individual nursing judgment and actions.
5. Maintaining competence in nursing.
6. Using informed judgment with individual competence as criteria in seeking consultation, accepting responsibilities, and delegating nursing responsibilities to others.
7. Participating in activities that contribute to ongoing development of the profession's body of knowledge.
8. Participating in professional efforts to implement and improve standards of nursing.
9. Participating in professional efforts to establish and maintain conditions of employment conducive to quality nursing care.
10. Participating in professional efforts to protect the public from misinformation and misrepresentation and to maintain the integrity of nursing.
11. Collaborating with members of health professions and others in promoting community and national efforts to meet public health needs.

American Nurses' Association. *Code for Nurses with Interpretive Statements.* Kansas City, MO, 1976.

INDEX